*HELP THEM TO COPE WITH*
*THE ALIENATION THEY WILL FEEL*
*GIVE THEM LOVE AND SUPPORT*
*ENCOURAGE THEM TO READ ANYTHING*
*GUIDE THEM IN DEVELOPING A SENSE OF HUMOR*
*GIVE THEM A CHANCE TO EXCEL*
**and the odds are—they will!**

# BELIEVE THE HEART:
## *Our Dyslexic Days*

*Elizabeth Fleming*

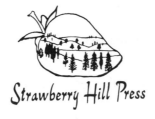

*Strawberry Hill Press*

Strawberry Hill Press
2594 15th Avenue
San Francisco, California 94127

Edited by Anne Griffiths

Acquisitions Editor: Jackie Dewey Everingham

Proofread by Diane Rae

Pasteup by Judith E. Merwin

Cover by Ku, Fu-sheng

Sketches by Ellanor Fleming

Backcover photo courtesy of *The Star-News*

Typeset by Cragmont/Ex-Press, San Francisco

Printed by Edwards Brothers Inc., Ann Arbor, Michigan

Manufactured in the United States of America

**Library of Congress Cataloging in Publication Data**

Fleming, Elizabeth, 1926-
    Believe the heart.

    Bibliography:p.
        1. Fleming, Elizabeth, 1926-    2. Dyslexia—
Patients—United States—Biography.  3. Dyslexic Children
—Education.  I. Title.
RC394.W6F57  1984    616.85'53    84-75
ISBN 0-89407-061-4

# DEDICATION

This book is dedicated to my family,
without whom there would have been no
story, and to Jackie Dewey, Ruth Pertel,
Peggy and Bertie Lippincott, and Meg Fleming,
who gave me the emotional support and
reassurance to write it. Special thanks
to my children, Elizabeth, Thomas, Ellanor,
George, and Richard who contributed so
much of their own time and energy to their
chapters, and to my mother, who provided
a place by the sea for me to write.

# TABLE OF CONTENTS

# INTRODUCTION

When my last child went off to college, it was suggested I write a book about my life as a hereditary dyslexic and how I raised five hereditary dyslexic children, who have all done well in higher education.

Elizabeth is a speech pathologist at the Frost Center, Rockville, Maryland.

Thomas is Director of the Law Library, United States Department of Commerce.

Ellie completed postgraduate work in architectural drafting.

My younger sons, George and Richard, are still in college. George is interested in systems analysis, and Richard has a B.S. in biology and is starting his masters in education.

Most hereditary dyslexics have a hard time learning to read. However, one can be a dyslexic and still know how to read. Dyslexics think in concepts and pictures instead of words. Until very recently, I didn't know that anyone thought in words. Can you imagine the problems that arise when an educator or parent who thinks in words tries to teach a child who thinks in pictures and concepts?

Unique spelling problems can persist throughout a dyslexic's life. While writing this book, I've encountered several— marriage/mirage, scared/scarred, routine/rotten. Marshall McLuhan's message/massage is another example.

My story as a self-educated hereditary dyslexic is told first, and then the children tell what they remember of their school days. Richard's is the longest, perhaps because his hereditary dyslexia was the most severe.

This is the story of six real people. I am writing the facts as well as I remember them. I have tried to keep the simple sentence structure of the dyslexic to help the reader enter into the world of dyslexia.

**Hereditary Dyslexia In One U.S. Family, 1856-1984**

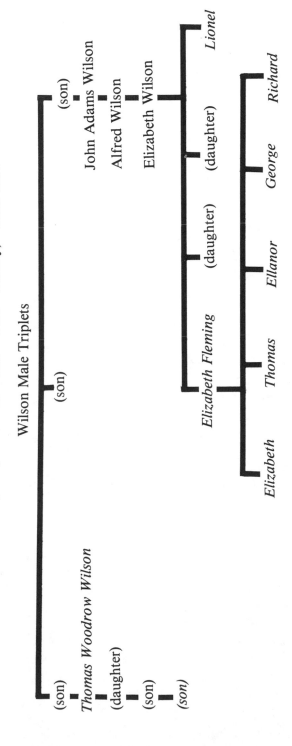

(Notes: The names in italics indicate hereditary dyslexia; the data are incomplete—only the author's family line is known in its entirety.)

# CHAPTER 1

## ON MY OWN: scared/scarred

My suitcase was packed. The day after Christmas, George, my husband, drove me to the hospital in Pittsburgh. Our marriage counselor, who was a physician, had made my reservations and they were in order. It's not that easy to sign yourself into a psychiatric hospital.

Once I was inside, three different psychiatrists interviewed me. Each one asked me to tell him the story of my life, which I did. And "Why did I want to sign myself into the psychiatric hospital?" Each time I answered, "For psychological testing."

I was determined to get this point straightened out once and for all. I wanted expert testimony that I was emotionally sound, and that I was *not* a "stupid little idiot." I had been called that when, as a child, I had difficulty learning to read. I wanted to prove to our marriage counselor, my husband, and the world that I was mentally and emotionally strong enough to take care of all five of my children. My husband wanted a divorce and custody of the children.

"Dummy" was another word used in my childhood for people like me. Today the word is *"dyslexic."* Years after my admission to the psychiatric hospital, all five of my children and I were diagnosed as hereditary dyslexics.

A definition I found years later states that *dyslexia* means "faulty reading." Twenty-three million Americans may have dyslexia to some degree. It is probably inherited, it occurs in the otherwise intelligent, it is more common in boys than in girls, and it is *never the same in two individuals*.

I was plenty scared that first day at the hospital when I was asked to sign a release that would authorize not only psychological testing and evaluation, but also any kind of physical treatment, including a lobotomy. My brain was more important to me than anything; it had taken so long to train.

I asked the doctor in as light and as steady a voice as I could muster, "I hope you would get another evaluation and consultant before you would do anything as drastic as that."

He answered, "Of course we would. The paper is just a formality." So I signed it.

I was then taken to the elevator, where I said goodbye to George. The elevator took the nurse and me to the ninth floor. We got out and walked down the corridor toward a door that was opened for us. Once over the threshold, we were locked in. The door slammed shut with a metal clank! I'll never forget that sound.

The nurse showed me around the floor, the TV room, the living room, the office, a few private rooms, and four wards. I was checked in at the office and then shown my bed and bureau in one of the wards. The nurse told me to change out of my clothes into a hospital gown and robe so that my clothes could be taken and marked. As soon as I was changed, I was to take a bath. The nurse showed me into the bathroom, helped me draw the bath, and then sat down to watch me bathe. I asked her why.

She said, "Rules."

This was the first time anyone had cared whether I drowned in a bathtub since I was a little child. There was a certain security in it. These people did care whether I lived or died.

When I started to let out the water, the nurse said, "You're not finished yet. You didn't wash your arms."

"You're just as fussy as a mother," I quipped back.

It was now dinner time. The other patients went across the hall for dinner. I felt quite left out. It was explained to me that I couldn't go into the hall without my day clothes. I wasn't sure that I would ever get them back again. A card table was set up for two in the living room and trays were sent over from the dining room. Another new girl had come in. She didn't have her day clothes either. Although we were introduced, we didn't talk much at first. She was younger than I, pretty, and about four months pregnant.

Then she began to cry. That brought me out of myself. I started to talk to her, realizing that here was someone feeling just about the same way I did. I felt very protective toward her, for my marriage trouble had started when I was three months pregnant. The thing that upset her the most was having to wear the hospital clothes and, as she pointed out, mine were a newer style than hers. I offered to trade with her. We did change clothes and she felt much better. And it certainly made me feel better to help her.

The first night I could not go to sleep for nearly two hours because a nurse came by every half hour and shined a flashlight in my face. Eventually I placed my head at the foot of the bed, where I could see out the window, and fell asleep.

By noon the next day my clothes had been returned and I could eat in the dining room with the other women. Nurses waited on the tables so they could keep track of how much you ate. I asked why.

Another patient replied, "One way to commit suicide is to starve yourself to death."

So it was a very bad sign not to eat.

The enormity of what I had done did not hit until the second day. I had signed myself into the hospital. I had wanted to prove that I was not stupid. Yet there I stood in the middle of a nut house, saying to myself, "Now you have done it! Maybe they were right, all those years ago, and maybe I am a 'stupid little idiot.'"

I was so frightened that for twenty-four hours I couldn't even go to the bathroom.

I sat in the recreation room, feeling very blue and down in the dumps, trying to make some sense out of all this nonsense.

I started talking to a girl who was looking through the bars at the window. I asked her, "What do you do for reassurance? How do you keep your mental balance?"

She responded, "Remember one thing. It's the nuts out there that put us in here."

We both laughed. It was good reassurance, and I needed all I could get.

It didn't take me long to see that no one else was there in the hospital for the same reason I was. Everyone else with whom I spoke had been committed, whereas I had signed myself in. Many had tried to commit suicide—using every means, from taking a light overdose of sleeping pills to swallowing lye. I had been depressed. I had been angry. But a general curiosity had always stood me in good stead. I always wanted to know what was going on. Suicide would be the farthest thing from my mind. I also found out that I was the only patient whose parents had been divorced.

When the realization hit me that I had no idea how to get out of the hospital, nor how long I would have to remain, I began to make up my own rules. That is one of the side joys of being in a psychiatric hospital; no one can do anything to frighten you any more.

Number one rule, for myself, would be to tell the *truth*, no matter what the psychiatrists or psychologists asked me. One concession I realized I was ready to make—only if I had to—was to give up God if that was what it was going to take to get me out of this isolated hell and back to my children. They were all under the age of twelve.

I had noticed a display case in the hospital craft room. Only two major shapes were on display—phallic symbols and Christian crosses.

When I asked the nurse why these were the only two forms on display, she answered, "They are the only two categories the patients seem to be interested in."

That bit of information registered. I wasn't likely to make clay figures look like phallic symbols but I might have decided to make a Christian statue or cross. Whoever set up that display case might feel that sex and religion were signs of mental illness. I would take note and stay away from both subjects. So I made a wooden stool for my children to stand on to reach the bathroom sink.

The awesome question was, "How long will I be locked up?" Our marriage counselor thought I would be there for six months. I still did not know why he had been so afraid I was losing my mind, or why he thought I might be suicidal.

I thought of my friend Dr. Nar's experience. He had been in a Japanese prisoner-of-war camp for four years. Remembering how he had come out and put those four years to good use made me realize that I could do it too, without losing my mind.

In hospital slang, I was classified under "husband trouble." The other main category was "mother trouble." When there were bull sessions, mothers were often discussed. But when the subject got too touchy, you would often hear, "Let's not talk dirty. Husbands are an easier subject to take."

I had been assigned to the ninth floor. The extremely disturbed were put on the seventh, the half-ways on the ninth, and the ready-to-be-released and the ready-to-crack again on the tenth. There was only one floor for men, the eighth; so they couldn't tell whether they were getting better or worse. Some of the men were taken out of there to be put in the state hospital, always in strait jackets.

One of the first things I had to conquer was fear. I mean real fear. In a psychiatric hospital you lose your identity. The first day you don't even have your own clothes on your back. Outside the hospital the day before, the person you felt you were, internally and externally, was a free citizen. You might have had problems, but so did everyone else. Now, today, you are locked up in a psychiatric hospital. One day you are a free adult, and the next day you are locked up and treated as a child that has just lost its mind. No, that's not fair—you are just treated as a child. But a mighty young one.

It took about three weeks to run through the entire psychological testing. When I was scheduled to start, I was delighted. It gave me something to do. The boredom in the hospital was excruciating. I was absolutely unafraid of testing.

After all, what could anyone do to punish me if I failed or didn't do well? I was already in a psychiatric hospital. And it would be fun to see how well I could do. Until that day I had always been very frightened of any kind of test. But no more!

The psychologist was pleasant and put me at ease immediately. He was calm and matter-of-fact about the testing. I must say, when some questions came up like, "Why is a fly like a tree?" or "Why is a book like a poem?" I asked myself, My stay depends on this?

I was given mazes to do, like the black-and-white ones that I had seen in the funny papers for years. I had not done one since I was a child. There I was, with pencil in hand, working my way through three sheets of them. I found, much to my amazement, that I could comprehend the entire maze and see the way out within seconds. At the end of my hospital stay I had to do a similar series. The doctor noted that it took me longer than the first series had done.

But by then I was certain I would be out of the hospital and so I didn't have to think as fast any more.

Boredom was the worst thing to fight. I had thought that one of the advantages of being in the hospital was that you would be able to see your psychiatrist every day. Forget it. I was there for two weeks before I was able to make an appointment with mine. Then she broke two appointments. I asked to speak to the second-in-command, Dr. Bro.

I told him about my being in the hospital for two weeks and not even seeing my psychiatrist. How, when an appointment was made, it was canceled.

"What are you trying to do to me? Test me for rejection, just to see how I will handle it?"

I was very angry at the hospital and at my psychiatrist and told him so. I also complained because I couldn't have a pass (as some of the other patients did) to get off the ninth floor and visit other parts of the hospital.

"I want to get out of here. I want to be at home with my children and the new baby," and I started to cry. "I have done everything I can do on my own. I've written down every dream I can remember and all my childhood history from the age of two. But there is no doctor to talk to. And the boredom is enough to drive me crazy.''

He gave me a pass to the library and was very kind. He gave me a pep talk.

''You want to make sure that you are in good shape to take care of your children. You don't want to be a neurotic mother. Stay here and finish the testing and you will always know that you have done the very best for your children—that is, to give them an emotionally healthy mother.''

I felt much more reassured and thanked him very much for his time. I asked him if he would be my psychiatrist, but he said he couldn't.

The hospital was a training hospital for young psychiatrists. The one assigned to me was a woman who had been born and raised in Sewickley, the same town I lived in. She had even gone to my church. I didn't find this out until a week later, when she finally made an appointment that she could keep. I saw her three other times.

One day, I saw my obstetrician, Dr. Pink, on the hospital ward and asked him, ''What are *you* doing here?''

''I'm the gynecologist and obstetrician for the women's ward,'' he answered, ''What are *you* doing here?''

I later told my psychiatrist how upset I was at seeing Dr. Pink. I felt as though I had lost face.

She said, ''You were upset! It took me two hours to quiet him down after seeing you in here.''

My first visitor was my friend Ann, from Sewickley. She gave me two books as a present, Paul Tillich's *The Courage to Be* and *The Human Spirit*, edited by Whit Burnett.

She said, ''I'm scared to death. I just came up in the elevator with two patients who had just had shock treatment. They were so out of focus.''

I could see that Ann was terrified, even though there had been nurses with the patients. She had never seen anything like that before. As a matter of fact, neither had I. I suppose, as a rule, the nurses kept such patients out of the halls until they became more coherent, so the rest of us wouldn't be frightened.

There had been one exception. One evening one of the teenagers on our ward was put in a private room. I walked past the room and looked in. One of my roommates stood talking to her. The teenager was terrified.

I asked, "What is wrong? What has happened?"

She had been given scopolamine, my roommate explained. "She can't forget the horror of trauma she blocked out for years. The drug will wear off soon, and she will forget; but in the meantime, she is terrified."

I went in to see if I could help.

"Try to think of something happy that happened to you in your life," we offered.

"I can't think of anything that did," she replied.

"Come on. Think of something. A vacation you once had. A trip to the beach," I coached.

"I can remember once being on a large inner tube, floating on a lake," she answered.

At last some memory had come to take her mind off her earlier family trauma. We helped her remember more of how it had felt to be floating safely, under the warm sun. Finally she went to sleep.

Getting acquainted at the hospital was just about the same as anywhere else. The dorms were like those at boarding school or camp. Basic personality doesn't change in the hospital. Some patients were thought to be real nuts when they came in sick; we felt the same way about them when they were discharged. I even complained to my psychiatrist about one woman who stayed in two weeks and was then released.

The doctor said, "Some of the patients we just patch up and let out. There isn't anything really to work with—no potential."

Others were delightful when you first met them, and even when they became "stark raving sane," as we put it, their personalities stayed the same.

By and large, the patients in the hospital had been hurt so badly during their lives that they had lost the will to fight.

One lady in her sixties had come to the hospital after she had gotten some false teeth that didn't fit her. That was the straw that had broken her back. She and I were scheduled to take our "Frankenstein tests" at the same time. (That was what they called the Funkenstein test on our hall.)

She and I were walking down the hall when she said, "Where are you going?"

I couldn't help myself; I said, "Crazy! Do you want to come along?"

She didn't laugh. She said, "Aren't you afraid?"

"Listen, I am so frightened, but you can't know what courage is until you know what real fear is."

With that she quieted, and we walked on down the hall together.

The Funkenstein test is given to see how you react to certain drugs—insulin, for example. We had to lie down on hospital beds, and a nurse and our psychiatrist stood by while we were injected with different hypodermic needles and our reactions were recorded. I recall saying that I felt as though I had just stopped running, after one of the shots. There was perspiration around my lips and my heart beat rapidly. I must have passed the test because I didn't hear any more about it.

The hospital staff tried to provide some kind of recreation. One night we had a dance with the men from the eighth floor. I thought of Arthur Murray's slogan, **Learn how to be popular—Learn how to dance**. The dance was the same as any one I had ever been to, the dancers as good or bad. But I had to laugh during one square dance. There we were, all patients trying to find our identities, but since there were not enough men the teacher made some of us put on green ties and be men. As if we didn't have enough problems already!

In the hospital everyone was kind. If you started to cry, someone would put a tissue in your hand, without saying a word. There was no problem with sexual attachment. No one had the energy for it. There was just tremendous concern and love for each other. We were all in this together.

One of the new girls who had been there before told me, "The trick in getting out of here is to express your anger."

The next day this tremendous feeling of anger rose up in me. I found a large blackboard in one of the rooms and wrote

on it all the four-letter words I could think of and some I
didn't think I knew. One of the very disturbed girls looked in
through the doorway and became frightened.

"You do that and they will lock you up in a padded cell."

"I don't give a damn," I answered back, "It would be
worth it."

Of course no one locked me up. I suspect the nurses were
glad to see me let out my anger at my husband.

I had always been a daughter, a sister, a wife, an
Episcopalian, a mother, but who was I? One book that Ann
had brought me, Tillich's *The Courage to Be*, was a
tremendous help to me, for it addressed itself to this very
problem. Stripped of all outward symbols, who are we?

Well, I did know my name was Elizabeth and I was born
June 25, 1926. That much I knew for certain.

Later Dr. Nar had kidded me, "That's right, just give them
name and serial number."

My minister came to see me the fourth week I was there. I
asked him why he hadn't told me it was so hard to be a
Christian. I remember his telling the story of the bishop
looking out his window at the beggar in the street and saying,
"There, but for the grace of God, go I."

I had decided that I would divorce George. It was the only
thing I could do.

My constant friend and confidant was God, in my prayers.
I had not worried about giving Him up; that would have been
a waste of energy, and I didn't have it to spare.

Two important spiritual insights came to me during that
period of confinement, while I was in hell, away from my
children for so long.

The first was that Jesus was giving me his example, "and he
suffered and was buried and descended into hell. The third day
he rose again and sat on the right hand of God." He had been
where I was.

The second insight came through active imagination. I saw
myself standing in a long line of people. It was dark, but I
could clearly see the people in line with me.

Finally I reached the head of the line. An old man in a
white robe, with a long white beard and white hair was

standing on the right, asking questions of each of us. At first I couldn't hear him; then it was my turn. He asked me this question: "What have you done with your life?"

I replied, "I have five lovely children."

He looked at me and said, "You were one of my children, too." He repeated, "What have you done with your life?"

I have not been able to answer that question, but I know it is an important one—perhaps the most important question I will ever be asked.

Three years earlier, an English minister had given us the laying-on-of-hands service at our church. He had said, if we didn't have anything physically wrong with us that we wanted healed, to come to the altar rail anyway if we had a spiritual request. I remember looking at the altar, and to the right I visualized the form of Jesus. I said, in prayer to Jesus, that I had known happiness and indeed was happy (I was married and had three children at the time), but that I didn't know what joy was, and that the readings in the Bible, and sermons and prayers, had led me to believe that Christian joy was something to have.

Little did I know then what I had done. I have since used the phrase, "You had better check it out with a lawyer before you put something into a prayer of request or petition." For to know joy you have to know sorrow. I had remembered the line in *The Brothers Karamazov*, "It's the great mystery of human life that old grief passes gradually into quiet joy." I knew it was important, but I didn't understand it at that time.

In Tillich's essay, "The Meaning of Joy," I found the original reference from John 16:20-22:

*Truly, truly, I say to you, you will weep and lament, but the world will rejoice; you will be sorrowful, but your sorrow will turn into joy.*

and from Psalm 126:5-6:

*May those who sow in tears reap with shouts of joy! He that goes forth weeping, bearing the seed for sowing, shall come home with shouts of joy, bringing his sheaves with him*

When I had first come into the hospital, I had felt like the Old Testament "My God is an angry God," and it was good to feel this—to be angry and to feel. Through the feeling of this passionate anger, coupled with the feeling of love, I realized that anger and love were not at opposite ends of a stick, but somehow formed a circle. And at the point where they met was passion, both physical and emotional passion. With passion, and with the ability to feel passion, one could know and feel compassion. *Compassion is empty without passion.*

On the day of my psychiatric evaluation and my personal interview with thirty-one members of the hospital staff, I was again reading Tillich. I was terribly excited about the essay. But my hospital psychiatrist, when I tried to talk to her about it, told me to stop unless I wanted them to think that I was crazy.

She didn't frighten me, I knew by then that I was all right. But it had taken every bit of ingenuity and honesty with myself to find that out.

When I entered the conference room, a doctor asked, "How do you feel about your marriage?"

"Unfulfilled," I replied.

They noted that. That was a satisfactory answer, and I was shortly told that I could leave the room again.

I asked one of the girls I knew slightly, who had been at the hospital when I first got there, "Do you notice any difference in me from the time I first came here to now?"

I expected her to say no, for I noticed no difference in myself.

Much to my surprise she answered, "Oh yes. You don't talk as fast." (To this day, when I get excited, I still talk too fast.)

I was discharged from the hospital with a clean bill of health. The hospital suggested a particular psychiatrist I might want to see during the period of my divorce and the adjustment to raising five children by myself. I would have a trained adult to whom I could talk.

I thought it was a good idea, but although it was pleasant enough for the first few visits, it turned into a nighmare! My divorce lawyer proved to be very weak and was constantly swayed by the stronger lawyer on the other side. I was thinking about changing lawyers and told my psychiatrist so.

"If you do that I will have you committed," he told me.

I was furious. I phoned Dr. Bro at the hospital and asked him what he would suggest I do. I also asked, "Why did the hospital choose that particular psychiatrist for me?"

He answered, "That doctor thinks slowly; you have a very fast mind. We thought you two might complement each other."

Dear God! It was the first time anyone had ever told me that I had a quick mind. I had heard as a child that I was "slow witted" or "dumb" because I couldn't talk until I was three-and-a-half. And when I couldn't read either, I thought that meant that my mind was slow. And now to hear I had a fast mind. No wonder it had bothered that psychiatrist when I talked fast. I knew what I was saying, but his own mind did not work fast enough to take it in. It didn't mean that my mind was better than his or that I was smarter, it just meant that my mind could receive information and think more rapidly than his could.

Dr. Bro told me of another psychiatrist, Dr. Joh. Because he had been a colleague of Dr. Nar's, I switched psychiatrists immediately. I then phoned my mother and asked her to come up and stay with me for a while. I had to get things straightened out. I needed her strength. She was the best fighter I knew. And I needed fighters.

My first visit to Dr. Joh was such a relief. He knew Dr. Nar and had spoken to him on the telephone about me. At the end of the hour he said, "You haven't cried enough."

And I started to cry.

"Go ahead and cry," he said.

"For how long?" I asked.

"Two days, if you like."

Dr. Joh suggested that my anxiety might have been caused by my feeling that, once I was divorced, I would be dependent on my mother. He wanted to see me again, after my mother's visit, to see how it had gone.

When my mother arrived, I hadn't yet found a good divorce lawyer. After hearing how much help my obstetrician, Dr. Pink, had been to me while I was pregnant, and how he had vouched for my sanity when I was in the hospital, Mother phoned him and asked him for the name of a good lawyer. He was most concerned and gave us the name of his own. Mother helped me change lawyers and then returned to Washington. She had been a tremendous help.

I went to see Dr. Joh again, for my last visit. We talked for an hour. My mother's visit had gone well, and I had a new lawyer who was as tough as nails. At the end of the session Dr. Joh said, "I find you normal, Mrs. Fleming, and in good mental health."

Those were the loveliest words I will ever hear.

"It's the first time anyone has ever told me so," I said.

Compassion was new to me and I could feel the tears welling up.

I had asked Dr. Joh to check my hospital records to find out what had been said. He told me that my husband had told the marriage counselor that he thought I would try to commit suicide, and that there was no other woman in his life. It was all a figment of my imagination, and I was hallucinating.

Wow, scary! He had lied. By then he was living with the other woman. (They were married right after our divorce.)

Dr. Joh asked me if what my husband had said bothered me.

I answered no, and I meant it. Nothing my husband said mattered any more.

Never tell a marriage counselor that you have read the Greek play *Medea* (the story of an unfaithful king whose wife, Queen Medea, murdered their two children for revenge). I had told my counselor that I thought Freud had missed something in not using *Medea* as a psychiatric tool, as he had used *Oedipus Rex*. Well, that was the end of me. I'll bet I am the first recorded case of "Medea complex."

I had told my husband, "Shape up or ship out"—an old military expression for "change your attitude or leave." But that, too, had been interpreted as a very bad sign. The counselor didn't know this military slang, and he had given it a deep Freudian meaning.

One very positive thing came out of having my records checked. I found out that I had a high I.Q.

So much for my dummy complex. It would have to go.

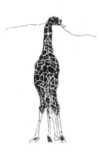

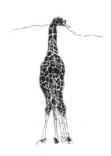

# CHAPTER 2

## WHAT IS DYSLEXIA?

Dyslexic: *A person with a problem with reading and spelling, usually of average intelligence or above, who does not respond to the usual teaching methods in reading or spelling.*

Some famous writers are believed to have been dyslexic, for example, Hans Christian Andersen, Agatha Christie, William Butler Yeats, and Gustave Flaubert. Other famous political, scientific, and cultural figures believed to have been dyslexic include Thomas Edison, George Patton, Auguste Rodin, and Albert Einstein.

Professionals in education and medicine tend to look at the word in different ways. The educator usually uses the word *dyslexic* to label any person who does not read well, regardless of the reason. The medical professional tends to use the word *dyslexic* to describe a person whose problem is hereditary.

Hereditary dyslexics have problems with reading and spelling, but in their cases the cause is a hereditary trait in the family. In our family, this trait can be traced back through my mother's family to my great-grandfather John Adam Wilson's first cousin, Woodrow Wilson. One of Woodrow Wilson's great-grandsons is a hereditary dyslexic, as are my brother and I, and all of my five children.

The description given by the Orton Dyslexia Society, a national organization devoted exclusively to helping individuals with dyslexia, includes the following:

1. Severe difficulty in learning and remembering the printed word or symbol.

2. Reversals of letters or improper letter sequence (e.g., *b* for *d*, *was* for *saw*).

3. Bizarre spelling errors.

4. Illegible handwriting.

5. Poor composition (difficulty putting words and sentences together).

Fortunately, very few people exhibit all of the characteristics of dyslexia, but dyslexics have enough in common to distinguish them as a group with unique educational needs.

Why have hereditary dyslexics been so harshly labeled with words like brain damage, minimal brain dysfunction, low I.Q.?

Are we afraid of that which is not average, that which is not usual?

When I was a child, hereditary dyslexics were called dumb or stupid. What was worse, *most of us believed it*. The educators had support for their statements—our low I.Q. test scores! If you can't read and write well, it is nearly impossible for you to take a written I.Q. test, least of all receive a decent grade.

My children used to pass the word to each other, "Take the test anyway. You get two hundred points for signing your name right."

In 1959, Dr. Knud Hermann, in his book *Reading Disability: A Medical Study of Word-Blindness and Related Handicaps*, wrote, "It would undeniably be a social advance if research into word-blindness would convince teachers...and prigs that defective spelling ability is not a sign of stupidity."

I did not learn to spell my name consistently correctly until I was in the fifth grade. At times it would come out with an *s* instead of a *z—Elisabeth*.

My brother and I had to repeat a grade, as did my older daughter and son, because of our poor reading skills. The word *dyslexia* was not introduced into our family vocabulary until 1966, when I was forty. My youngest son, Richard, was in the first grade, and a child psychiatrist pointed out the reason for our trouble, or rather gave it a name—hereditary dyslexia. It was a relief to know.

The frustration at being bright and not being able to learn in the same manner as your peers can become nearly unbearable. You have two choices. You can fight back and try to prove that you aren't dumb, which is nearly impossible to do, for the common attitude is that any dummy can learn to read. Or you can become lethargic ("lazy") and take on an I-don't-care attitude. Neither is good, but you have to cope in some manner.

It has been my experience that there have been other qualities that *some* hereditary dyslexics have that are not usually mentioned.

1. They think in pictures and concepts, not in words.

2. They are clairsentient (feel the emotions of other people).

3. They have faster minds than average people.

4. They speak rapidly.

5. They have the ability to discuss concepts, without becoming emotional about them.

6. They become emotional about some words and want to pin down the meanings and origins of them.

7. They have creative thinking and problem-solving abilities (when tested appropriately)—abstract thinking talents.

8. They have trouble with written languages that use alphabets—but not with Chinese characters and pictorial written languages (ideograms).

9. They are good at sign language (in which signs substitute for spoken words) but not at finger spelling (in which the hands are used to indicate letters).

When asked questions, hereditary dyslexics answer them differently than average people. They give conceptual rather than simply straight-line verbal responses. They don't see answers in words, but in causality. They automatically (in some cases) think of answers at many different levels of awareness—all at the same time.

A friend, Jack Lauritzen, a solid-state physicist, once told me that he had the idea for a paper he had to write and present, but that he hadn't put it into written form.

I asked him about the process, and he answered, "An idea or concept—I have to take it from the nebulous, non-dimensional space to the linear. To the written word in English. Like a choo-choo train, left to right, on a straight line."

It was hard for him to do, and he wasn't dyslexic.

Dyslexics tend to answer questions while thinking aloud. This can be very confusing to the person asking the question—unless that person is another dyslexic. At the same time, the fact that they seldom use adjectives or adverbs can make their answers seem clipped. If one does not listen carefully, the whole point of what they say can be missed. It slips out so quickly.

One theory is that the average person trains one side of the brain to gather and tabulate information, and that the other side of the brain monitors and modulates extraneous information of sight and sound to prevent "overloading" of the brain. The hereditary dyslexic processes information into both sides of the brain and therefore can be subject to temporary "overloading." A child's reaction to this is often to stare out of the school window or stop listening—to tune out for a while.

This bilateral control is often misinterpreted, by those not familiar with the phenomenon, as a *lack* of control.

What may seem to others to be scattered and disorganized thinking can, to the hereditary dyslexic, make perfectly good sense—be actually under control, but in the hereditary dyslexic's own frame of reference. This may not only work well for him in daily living, but also lead to valuable moments of creativity and innovation.

The final word is not in yet on whether the thing that separates the functions of the two sides of the brain in the average person is a gate or a guard, an advantage or a limitation. Maybe its absence is what allows the dyslexic to grasp more complicated concepts as a whole, even though spelling may never be easy, and the individual letters of the alphabet may be a mystery in childhood.

In some cases, the hereditary dyslexic sees symbols on the printed page or on the blackboard as floating and having no top, bottom, left, or right. The *b* in *boy* doesn't come through as a two-dimensional symbol, but as a three-dimensional one. It's perceived as an odd-shaped ball that the hereditary dyslexic's brain plays with—turning and throwing it in the air. No wonder the dyslexic gets mixed up—while floating in the air, the *b* can look like a *p*, a *d*, or a *q*.

The concept of dyslexia can be better comprehended with an example of a dyslexic's written language. In the following example, the errors are not typing ones.

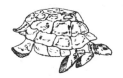

John Fleming
Eckerd College
P. O. Box 333
St. Petersburg, Fl 33733

E.R. Fleming
642 Ocean Lane #5
Imperial Beach, Ca 29232

May 11.1982

Dear E.R.Fleming

This is a note of expanses for the summer term of 1982. The total amount is 1842.50 (look at list below). The two class I will be tacking are S.E.M. tenecs and I hope Chemistry, if not Chemistry I will be tacking some ather class.

list of expanses)

|     |                    |           |
| --- | ------------------ | --------- |
| a)  | Reat for 3 mouns   | $502.50   |
| b)  | Food for 10 weeks  | $350.00   |
| c)  | Tuition for 2 class| $990.00   |
|     | Totel              | $1842.50  |

I would like at this time to confast to the missus of $300.00. This mony was to be used in forthering me voic. But I used it in gating a bike $200.00, the remaber was used in my food bugat.

Im in date to you for this mony. I will not be abal to pay you back intil the end of Aug. 1982. I hope you uderstaned.

Love

John Richard Fleming

My son, John Richard Fleming, believes the dyslexic brain can be explained as follows:

**The average person, who thinks in words, takes a new word, or "given direction," and puts it in one pocket of the brain. The hereditary dyslexic, who thinks in concepts, not words, puts the information in many different conceptual pockets, because the information might be pertinent to or indicative of many different concepts.**

**An example: A phrase such as Shut up! would come to the average person as a command. But the hereditary dyslexic would file the information Shut up! under many other conceptual categories, such as, Shut-open, Shut-down, Shut-close, Shut-lock, and Up-down, Up-above, Up-sky.**

Richard is not implying that this is caused by the use of one side of the brain versus the other side, but rather by a bilateral (two-sided) organization versus a unilateral (one-sided) organization of the brain. (Sandra Witelson referred to the same phenomenon in the title of her article in *Science*, "Developmental Dyslexia: Two Right Hemispheres and None Left.")

I feel that hereditary dyslexia is a progressive hereditary trait, one that is increasing in the human population. More and more dyslexics are diagnosed every year. In the United States, an estimated 10 percent of the children entering kindergarten are being diagnosed dyslexic. It is a phenomenon that has been identified in more than twenty countries.

In these days of growing anxiety that modern man may not be able to keep up with the information explosion and technological advances made during this century, I suggest that man need not fear. Perhaps hereditary dyslexics are the new breed of man, an evolutionary species that does not live in a world of up-down, right-left, but rather in the multidimensional or nondimensional world of space.

Can this be called the Age of Dyslexia?

The geneticist Dr. Ruth Pertel wrote to me: "The major problem seems to be the way dyslexics are viewed by others, especially when they don't acquire certain tools that are common (such as reading and writing), until later in their development. So far no studies in any detail have been made about just what the dyslexic is acquiring as tools during this period."

Manuel Garcia Espita, a professor at Autonomous University of Baja California, Mexico, wrote in a letter to me: "It is commonly and rightly believed that a picture is worth a thousand words. Therefore, while non-dyslexics get *caught up* in words, dyslexics move ahead in pictures. To say that dyslexics are dumb is like saying that pictures do not exist. Science has put forth vital information in pictures. Therefore, denying dyslexics is denying science, art, and logic."

To this day, spelling is very difficult for me. As an example, two years after my experience in the psychiatric hospital I wrote a letter to Bentz Plageman, whose article I had read in the *Saturday Evening Post*.

The article described a hospital staff's insensitivity toward some paraplegic men's feelings of vulnerability and isolation. I cannot yet pick out the spelling mistakes that appear in this letter.

Bentz Plageman
c/o The Saturday Evening Post
Philadelphia 5, Pennsylvania

Dear Mr. Plageman,

I injoyed your article, "They Think We Have The Evil Eye." Particularly the view taken by the paraplegic in his reference to "taboo" and "socieites reject the deformed." I can't help but agree with him. I can not speak for society but I can for myself.

As a child and carried on into my late twenties. I was afraid of holloween. The masks that people wore frightened me. Only now do I realize what it was. I was afraid what might be behind the masks. In movies such as *The Hunch Back of Noter Dome* I was terrified when I saw his face for the first time.

I now find relief and laughter in movies about werwolfs, vampire, etc. Because when I see those faces now I realize that I am looking at my own subconcious. In the movie *Sparticus* I adentified with the woman who has leperasy. The mythical or taboo relationship between leperassy and insanity must be very close. When I was ill (suffering from acute infuriority complex and hospitalized for five weeks) I felt so ugly that to see it on the schreen was a relief (lepresy).

So I can't help but sympathize with those people who project themselves, and we all do, when they see a crippled person. They don't want to admit to themselves that they are emotionally crippled so they must reject the person who is crippled. Does this make sence to you? Most people are so afraid to admit that there is anything wrong with themselves.

Most Sincerely,

Elizabeth Fleming

# CHAPTER 3

## FAMOUS PEOPLE BELIEVED TO HAVE BEEN DYS-LEXIC

One of the most reassuring things I ever came across was that Albert Einstein (1879-1955) was thought to be a dyslexic. While researching a paper I wrote, "Einstein and Dyslexia," I read in Ronald Clark's book, *Einstein: The Life and Times*: "The one feature of his childhood about which there appears no doubt is the lateness with which he learned to speak. Even at the age of nine he was not fluent ... His parents feared that he might be subnormal, and it has even been suggested that in his infancy he may have suffered from a form of dyslexia."

Einstein's teachers told his father that he was "mentally slow, unsociable, and adrift forever in his foolish dreams."

It encouraged me to read that Einstein wrote that he thought his backwardness had its compensations.

"I sometimes ask myself, how did it come that I was the one to develop the theory of relativity? The reason, I think, is that a normal adult never stops to think about problems of space and time. These are things which he has thought of as a child. But my intellectual development was retarded, as a result of which I began to wonder about space and time only when I had already grown up. Naturally, I could go deeper into the problems than a child with normal ability."

It was probably a great help to Einstein that his father, Hermann, and his uncle Jakob had a small electrochemical works. This family business undoubtedly stimulated Einstein's interest in electricity.

I read that his uncle Jakob would talk with him and tell him stories. "Algebra is a merry science," Uncle Jakob would say. "We go hunting for a little animal whose name we don't know, so we call it $x$. We bag our game, we pounce on it and give it its right name." Later, when Einstein attempted to explain the theory of relativity to nonmathematicians, he would fall back on Uncle Jakob's analogies, only this time using elevators, trains, and ships.

Another uncle, Casar Koch, gave him a model steam engine. It was to Uncle Casar that Einstein, when he was sixteen, sent the outline of the imaginative ideas from which his special theory of relativity was developed. He proposed to tackle one of the most hotly disputed scientific subjects, the relationship between electricity, magnetism, and ether (that hypothetical, nonmaterial entity presumed to fill all space and to transmit electromagnetic waves.)

Einstein loathed his early, German school experiences. Not until 1895, when his family moved to Switzerland, did he have anything good to say about school. At the age of sixteen, he went to the cantonal school at Aarau. Here, teaching resembled university lectures rather than high-school instruction. Here Einstein was introduced to the outer mysteries of physics by a first-class teacher, August Tuchmid. For the first time, he enjoyed learning at school.

Einstein received the 1921 Nobel Prize in physics "for the photoelectric law and his work in the domain of theoretical physics."

In his book, *Ideas and Opinions, a Mathematician's Mind*, Einstein answered questions put to him by Hadamard, a scholar who was conducting a psychological survey of mathematicians to determine their mental processes during work.

*My Dear Colleague:*

*In the following, I am trying to answer in brief your questions as well as I am able...*

*The words or the language, as they are written or spoken, do not seem to play any role in my mechanism of thought. The psychical entities which seem to serve as elements in thought are certain signs and more or less clear images which can be "voluntarily" reproduced and combined...*

*This combinatory play seems to be the essential feature in productive thought—before there is any connection with logical construction in words or other kinds of signs which can be communicated to others.*

Some people are put off by the way dyslexics spell, and by their mistakes in punctuation and grammar when putting the written word down on paper. Because of these errors, many people jump to the conclusion that the dyslexic is stupid or slow.

But William Butler Yeats (1865-1939) never could spell or punctuate, according to his memoirs. Yet this famous Irish poet and dramatist has been judged by many to be the greatest twentieth century poet in the English language. Yeats wrote *The Land of Heart's Desire*, *The Countess Kathleen*, and *Deidre*, as well as many other works.

Yeats's father, John Butler Yeats, a famous painter, read aloud to his son for many years, and this may have been a contributing factor in helping a fine mind develop. In 1923, William Butler Yeats won the Nobel Prize in literature.

Many statues by Auguste Rodin (1840-1917), the French sculptor, are on display all over the world. Among the better known are *The Thinker* and *Hand of God*.

His father complained that he had an idiot for a son. When Rodin won an honorary degree from Oxford University at age sixty-seven, spelling and arithmetic were still difficult for him.

Hans Christian Andersen (1805-1875), the Danish poet, novelist, and writer of fairy tales, including such classics as *The Ugly Duckling, The Red Shoes*, and *The Snow Queen*, was criticized by one of his peers, C. Molbeck. In reviewing one of Andersen's books, Molbeck wrote, "When will such a prolific writer, already quite well known in his native country, learn to write his mother tongue correctly?"

Paul Ehrlich (1854-1915), the German bacteriologist, is remembered as a pioneer in the fields of hematology, immunology, and chemotherapy. He discovered the first cure for syphilis, popularly referred to as Doctor Ehrlich's Magic Bullet.

But he was so bad in German composition that he almost didn't graduate from preparatory school. He had terrible difficulty in taking written examinations, and his thesis for his medical degree was almost all in soneone else's handwriting, with added notes (with many spelling mistakes) by Ehrlich.

In her autobiography, Agatha Christie (1891-1976), beloved mystery writer, creator of dapper detective Hercule Poirot, author of sixty-eight novels and a hundred short stories, wrote that she "was an extraordinarily bad speller," and had "remained so until this present day."

She was known as the "slow one" of the family. No one treated her unkindly because of this. She accepted that it was true. She was slow—and went right on writing best sellers, *The Murder of Roger Ackroyd, And Then There Were None*, and *Witness for the Prosecution.*

Harvey Cushing (1869-1939), the brain surgeon, won a Pulitzer Prize for his biography of Sir William Osler.

But he had great difficulty in spelling. After he had won his medical degree, he sent in an application for a teaching chair at Yale University that had some of the words misspelled.

Because of the embarrassment most dyslexics suffer during their childhood, they try to hide their dyslexia. They don't want the world to know.

One of the rare authors who has written about being dyslexic under her real name is Eileen Simpson. She is a psychotherapist. In her book, *Reversals: A Personal Account of Victory over Dyslexia*, she tells how terrible it was to feel "dull-witted" for so long in her younger life.

She was married to John Berryman, the poet, for eleven years. She wrote him a note early in their love affair

*Dear*

*Time for olny a hurried note. M. and children well. Swimming every day despite gary skies. Tomorrow we calabrent M's birthday. See you Thursday.*
*In haste*
*Love*

John knew at once what was the matter. He said, "Your errors are not ordinary spelling errors. Hasn't anyone told you you have dyslexia?"

Simpson wrote: "It was a moment before I felt the swelling-up of pure joy. My affliction had a name!" And she repeated it—"lysdexia,"—an example of how some dyslexics transpose letters.

In her book, Simpson quotes Gustave Flaubert's niece, Caroline Commanville who wrote in "Souvenirs Intimes" about her famous uncle's troubles in learning to read: "Having made a strenuous effort to understand the symbols he could make nothing of, he wept giant tears . . . ."

In his youth, he was able to memorize much of *Don Quixote* by heart because a kind neighbor would recite it to him.

Other famous people who benefited from being read and recited to were Hans Christian Andersen, whose father read him Wolberg's plays and *The Arabian Nights*, Thomas Edison, Woodrow Wilson, and George Patton.

Thomas Edison's mother read to him from Gibbon, Shakespeare, and Dickens. This brilliant inventor (1847-1931), who gave the world the telegraph, the telephone, the phonograph, and the electric light bulb, and took out over thirteen hundred patents, was judged to be mentally ill by his teacher. So his mother (who had been a school teacher) got angry, took him out of school, and said she would teach him herself.

When he was much older, Edison wrote in his diary that his father thought he was stupid. Edison said he could never get on well at school and was always at the foot of the class.

Woodrow Wilson (1856-1924), president of Princeton University and, later, president of the United States and founder of the League of Nations, is said to have been unable to recite the alphabet until he was nine. His older sisters and his parents often read to him because he didn't learn to read until he was eleven. However, even in his early school years, he was a superior speechmaker.

George Patton (1885-1945), the U.S. Army general, earned a reputation during World War II as an outstanding leader. His nickname was Old Blood-and-Guts.

Because of his troubles in learning to read, his father had kept him out on their ranch and read to him instead of sending him to grade school. Young George went off to boarding school when he was twelve.

He never did learn to read very well; but fortunately he had an extraordinary memory and was able to get through West Point by memorizing whole lectures and texts, which he would recite in class word-for-word. He also loved poetry and composed some poems himself.

Nelson Rockefeller (1908-1979) was one of the rare famous people who admitted in public to being dyslexic. He would explain, when he sometimes transposed words or made other slips of the tongue, "That's just my dyslexia."

He always had difficulty reading, but he could conduct press conferences in three languages and read speeches—though he sometimes had to rehearse them six times, have the script prepared in large type, and have sentences broken into segments and long words broken into syllables.

He was vice-president of the United States under President Gerald Ford and governor of New York for four terms. He also held positions under Presidents Roosevelt, Truman, and Eisenhower.

Here is some advice from Nelson Rockefeller for dyslexics, particularly children, which appeared in *TV Guide*.

Based on my own experience, my message to dyslexic children is this:—Don't accept anyone's verdict that you are lazy, stupid, or retarded. You may very well be smarter than most children your age. Just remember that Woodrow Wilson, Albert Einstein and Leonardo da Vinci also had tough problems with their reading. You can learn to cope with your problem and turn your so-called disability into a positive advantage.

Dyslexia forced me to develop powers of concentration that have been invaluable throughout my career in business, philanthropy and public life . . . .

Looking back over the years, I remember vividly the pain and mortification I felt as a boy of 8, when I was assigned to read a short passage of Scripture at a community vesper service during summer vacation in Maine and did a thoroughly miserable job of it.

I know what a dyslexic child goes through—the frustration of not being able to do what other children do easily, the humiliation of being thought not too bright when such is not the case at all.

My personal discoveries as to what is required to cope with dyslexia could be summarized in these admonitions to the individual dyslexic:

Accept the fact that you have a problem—don't just try to hide it.

Refuse to feel sorry for yourself.

Realize that you don't have an excuse—you have a challenge.

Face the challenge.

Work harder and learn mental discipline—capacity for total concentration—and

Never quit!

# CHAPTER 4

## MY CHILDHOOD

The word "dummy" was one of the early taunts of my childhood. But I also remember how we played: murder-in-the-dark, blind-man's-bluff, king-of-the-mountain, and hide-and-seek.

I used to plant grass outside my playhouse because it grew so fast. One week, and you could see the blades of grass. A rewarding short-term goal, but in those days I didn't know that was what you called it.

I spent the first year of kindergarten on the East Coast, in Alexandria, Virginia, where I had been born. The classroom was so big—I never saw who was at the head of my table.

The following year, my family moved to Coronado, California. I repeated the afternoon kindergarten and loved it. We played, sang songs, and built houses out of large wooden blocks.

I moved up to the morning kindergarten the next semester. We played with numbers and alphabet pictures. I thought I would never get into first grade. The first graders used to taunt us, "Kindergarten-babies, kindergarten-babies!"

I did make it to first grade. Reading was easy. I was good at reading pictures. I just memorized "Jack and Jill ran up the hill." I sometimes got *house* and *home* mixed up because both words were printed under the same picture.

I sat at the "first table" in first grade. I was smart. One day the teacher found out I had told a fib. I would come in late to school because I played on the park merry-go-round. I told her I had been to the doctor. As a punishment, she put me down at the "dumb table," number five. I was totally humiliated and ashamed. If you are bad, you can't sit with the good students. You sit with the dumb ones—the ones that can't read. This was my first taste of discrimination.

In the second grade we had tables to ourselves. They were great, and I was doing all right. But one day the teacher stopped at my desk while I was writing and explained to me that I had to stop writing with my left hand and use my right hand.

"See the light coming through the window?" she said. "If you write with your left hand, a shadow will fall on your paper. The windows are placed so that all the children will have good light when they use their right hands."

It sounded logical to me, so I changed hands.

By the third grade I knew I was in the dumb section.

The teacher told me, "If you can memorize one hundred prepositions by the end of the year, I will pass you to the fourth grade."

I did memorize—"around, about, above, across, after, against, amidst..." But I did not understand the concept of what a preposition is all about until I was in my forties. Put a desk *in* a room. Stand *in front of* it. Now walk *toward* it. Walk *around* it. Stand *on top of* it. Crawl *under* it. I was so excited. I ran across the street and told my neighbors. Bless them. They listened.

How often do we let children talk about what they are thinking, instead of telling them what to talk about? *Know* is such a relative word.

My comforts were ice cream, Saturday matinees, and "Big-Little" children's books. They weren't into prepositions and adjectives.

In the fourth grade one of the girls asked me, "What boy do you like best?" I answered, "I don't like any boy, but if I did, it would be the one who sits in the first seat in the fifth row."

In the fifth grade the spelling list was so hard—"elephant, island..." I couldn't memorize the spelling of twenty words. My teacher caught me cheating five times. She made me stand up in front of the class and tell them that I had cheated and what a bad girl I was. I've never cheated again. I learned my lesson.

Later, remembering that time, I wrote a poem.

### FLASHBACK

I found myself crying this morning:
So much to learn, no one to teach me.
The delights of the mind,
the excitement of knowing,
were not to be mine.
Taunts at school—"You dummy!"
"Kindergarten-baby!"

"This girl was cheating!":
I could not remember the way to spell the words
so I wrote them on my arm.
I wanted to be bright
like the other children.

"Go take off that party dress!
You can't wear that!"
I wanted to look pretty at school.
So I changed—to another party dress.
And another, another.
Until there were five.
"I'll give you something to look pretty about!"
She whipped my ankles with a switch.

I still remember when I try to think of myself
as bright and pretty.

During the sixth grade I fell in love with Earl Brix. He was in the smart section. At last I was motivated. I wanted to get into his section of the class. I don't remember the subjects I had, but I know I got six A's. I wrote in my diary, "J'amo E.B."—a friend had taught me that code.

In the seventh grade, I began to look at the pictures in the newspaper. One day I asked my teacher, "What does it mean, 'the war in Spain?'"

The teacher said, "It doesn't count. We fought the First World War to end all wars."

That was the end of that subject. No new information. What good does it do to learn how to read?

In the eighth grade I did learn some new information, and the sense of mental isolation I had was lifted. A young man in the Civilian Conservation Corps came to our classroom and gave us a lecture on dinosaurs.

He was a former student of a marvelous math teacher we had—she was old, strict, and loved mathematics. His lecture gave me a sense of the vastness of the earth's history. Until then, teachers had just talked about California history—starting with the Spanish missionary system—and United States government. With the exception of my poor reading skills, I was average. I even won third prize in a track competition for broad jumping. My family congratulated me and then asked me to stop doing it. It was considered unlady-like.

I wasn't considered a good artist as a child because I couldn't stay within the lines. But in the eighth grade I had a real art teacher. The New York World's Fair (1939) was on. Its logo took my fancy, and I drew it in charcoal. Then we worked on batiks (with dyes and wax). I even did a flower picture with watercolors that looked like an oil painting.

I took all of my work home to show my mother. She said, "It is very nice, dear." Mother wasn't into encouraging or discouraging her children.

A friend of my mother suggested that I be sent as a boarder to the Bishop's School for girls in La Jolla, California, so that I "might be exposed to a larger environment" when I started high school.

It was expected that I would marry young, as my mother had. Mother was not in favor of higher education.

She had often reassured me, when I had felt bad about being so dumb in reading, "It doesn't matter if you can't read. It doesn't pay a woman to be too bright." But she was in favor of my going to Bishop's.

When I entered the Bishop's School as a boarder in the ninth grade, the headmistress thought my handwriting was poor. She gave me lessons in printing.

The art teacher was superb. She was German and spoke with an accent, "Don't paint like ze penny postcard."

In English class we learned about the plays of Shakespeare, and I drew sketches of the leading characters. I used geometric figures for the king and queen—and just made the same forms, smaller, for the court figures.

I discovered algebra, too, and loved it—the search for the unknown $x$. Our algebra teacher gave us a lecture I have never forgotten. We had all been restless and talking in chapel. She said, "None of you knew enough to afford *not* to listen to the speaker. I am not a member of a church, but assure you that, in my experience, anything you ask for sincerely of God that does not involve someone else, will happen." She dared us to try it, as an experiment.

I used to say of one boy from grade school, "I hate him inside and out."

I prayed that I would no longer feel that way. It worked!

I received an F in Old Testament studies. I have never forgotten the names of the books in the Bible, nor the stories, but I just couldn't remember their order.

In my sophomore year, in 1941, my roommate's birthday was on December 7. Her family came down from Los Angeles and took us out for a party. While we were seated at the hotel table, the waiter came over and told us, "Pearl Harbor has been bombed!"

That was the end of a chapter in my life. My mother's family worried about us, living on the West Coast with the fear of Japanese bombings and with air-raid drills going on constantly. Within three months, they sent mother railroad tickets for all of us to come East and stay with them at their farm, Riverridge, in Franklin, Pennsylvania.

The trip East was wild. To get us all packed was a major undertaking. There were three girls, brother Lionel, Mother, Miss Waters, and Chips, our dog. Miss Waters, our governess, always traveled like England's Queen Mary. Mother solved the luggage problem by crossing the border, to Tijuana, Mexico, and buying large straw baskets—two for each of us. They were very colorful and sturdy, with bright, woven flower designs. We children were allowed to pack one basket each with our treasures. We were assured that anything that didn't fit would be waiting for us when we returned after the war. We didn't have much to pack because of the warm California climate— no heavy coats.

At nine in the morning we were at the San Diego train station. The dog was in the baggage department, and the rest of us were waiting at the front of the train, ready to board. Some circus cars were attached to the rear of the train, and the conductor, on seeing us with our Mexican bags, told my mother in a loud voice, "Please move your group to the rear; the circus cars are at the back of the train." Mother assured him that we were not part of the circus, but I'm sure we looked like it, with our Mexican baskets and long faces.

Franklin was quite a shock to me. It was so quiet. I kept missing something—but it took me two weeks to realize that it was noise. Coronado had been noisy! We used to wait until the noise of airplanes overhead had passed to make sure a plane had not crashed. The destroyers and battleships in the bay were constantly coming and going with their shrill whistles, *whop whop whop whop*. Some nights you could hear the bosun whistle, *swi swi swi*, and the bosun saying, "Now hear this! Now hear this!..."

We children were enrolled in Franklin Public School. I was now in the second semester of my sophomore year. I had no trouble with my class in ancient history; I had studied it my freshman year at Bishop's. Latin II was another thing—the teacher was not as good as the one at Bishop's, and we had a different textbook.

In Franklin everybody in high school went steady. My steady beau was Bill Eggbeer. He was a year ahead of me and he helped me with Latin—*Caesar's Wars*. Spelling in Latin was not a problem for me because it was straightforward—it sounded the way it was spelled. But I had trouble remembering the vocabulary.

Bill was also a good dancer. One night we went to a movie in which a song was sung, *Arthur Murray Taught Me Dancing in a Hurry*. I asked Bill, "Who is Arthur Murray?" He answered, "The greatest teacher of ballroom dancing in the world."

The following year, I went off to boarding school—this time the Shipley School in Bryn Mawr, Pennsylvania. I was tested, and placed in the college preparatory section because of my background in mathematics (B and C grades), even though my English, spelling, and reading were way behind. By then I had a real dummy complex. I kept reassuring myself, "It-doesn't-matter-if-I'm-dumb."

English was a nightmare. The teacher announced on the first day of school, "Everyone who does good work will get a C. Anyone who does exceptional work will receive a B. Anyone who does work as well as I can will receive an A." I got an F. Trying to learn French was ridiculous. There was no way that I could make sense out of the spelling and all of the exceptions. One day we were reading from a new French primer. I was asked to read first. I couldn't make heads or tails of it. None of the words were spelled the way they sounded. The girl sitting next to me was then assigned the same paragraph. She read it in French, then translated it into English, "Once upon a time there were three bears. They lived in the forest."

With that I laughed and couldn't stop. The teacher sent me to the study hall. If I had only had one clue that it was the story of the three bears, I could have faked it—I could have recited it by heart. F in French.

My roommate that first year was Phyllis Murray. She and her sister Jane were boarders. They were the twin daughters of Kathryn and Arthur Murray. They also had just left California.

Jane's roommate, Gerry Taylor (an undiagnosed dyslexic), also had trouble getting good grades, but she tutored me through chemistry that first year. She took her class before mine and filled me in on what the teacher was going to talk about. Through her help and with some outside reading, I received a B in chemistry. Chemistry uses a lot of algebra, and I found the equations fun and easy. But it wasn't exciting.

Happy Fitler was a day pupil in our class. She later married Nelson Rockefeller. In all there were twenty-four girls in our class from all over the country. No boys.

That summer Mother took our family to Jamestown, Rhode Island. Families worried about polio every summer, and Jamestown, an island, had never had a polio case reported. I spent the summer as a volunteer for the Newport Navy Hospital Red Cross. Most of the boys were off to war.

The following year I was back at the Shipley School, with new teachers. Phyllis Murray was still my roommate, and Jane Murray and Gerry Taylor were our suite-mates. We were now seniors. I was still exchanging comic books, movie star books, magazines, and an occasional *Redbook* with a junior.

My English teacher complimented me on how well I was doing for someone with an I.Q. of 98. Come to think of it, when you can't read well and can't spell, that is a fairly respectable I.Q.

Perhaps the realization that I was doing better than was expected was one of the reasons I didn't advance myself past reading comic books and women's magazines. I liked the pictures and simple sentence structure and the imaginative stories. It never dawned on me that I could do better scholastically. Hadn't I been told that my I.Q. was 98—that I was doing the best that could be hoped for? All this confirmed the negative image I had of myself. I felt it was realistic. Only in these last few years has the emotional effect of that negative image become clear.

In English class we read Shakespeare's *Othello* and *A Midsummer Night's Dream*. When asked to read in class, I apologized for my poor reading, but the teacher asked me to go on because she liked the way I read the character. Earlier that year we had read *Beowulf*, which is in Old English. It was easier to read because the words sounded the way they were spelled.

The teacher gave us an assignment—to write a four-page paper on something that had happened to us. I wrote a story about what had happened to me in California during the summer before the war. Jane corrected the spelling for me. I got a B. Jane later told me, "The teacher discussed your paper in my class. She said that it was well written because the story was about a fourteen-year-old girl and the dialogue was true to the age of the character."

My senior year French teacher (bless her!) said that she would give Gerry and me a D-minus and allow us to graduate—if we could pass a test on how to read and order from a French menu. It was a make-up test. We had both flunked the original final, even after two years of trying.

Physics was the exciting course for me. It was a whole new world of laboratories, experiments, measures, and weights. It showed how the world worked, with laws and theorems. I loved it. I helped Phyllis with her lab work. She got a B in the class, and I received a C. I tended to transpose the numbers. I would write a *6* when I meant a *9*, or invert them when reading.

The physics teacher had said, "The atom is the basis of everything and you'd better remember that if nothing else." Sure enough, this was a question on the final exam. "Is the atom the basis of everything?" I wrote *no*.

By then the discipline of physics had trained my mind well enough that I felt it was impossible to answer the question *yes*, when it could not be proven that it was true.

But the teacher was good. He had taught me how to think. Like so many other people, I did not find out about the splitting of the atom until after the bombing of Hiroshima.

I had not been able to continue art at Shipley because it was not part of the college preparatory curriculum. However, when I wanted to go on with physics and mathematics, the counselors advised me not to do so because my grades were not strong enough.

During my last year at Shipley, I went to Philadelphia and took an all-day, comprehensive aptitude evaluation test. I didn't do well in art. The test was based on symmetry (as in Greek and Roman art) and not asymmetry (as in the art of the Orient). Modern art was not included in the testing at all.

My interest in medicine showed up. (The field of psychiatry was not included; it was too new.) Nursing was suggested as a possibility.

The one thing I scored very highly in was creative writing. The counselor gave the assignment, "Write what you would do to send information to another town if all the known forms of communication, such as telephone, telegraph, cars, and trains, were not working."

I asked him, "Does spelling count?" He answered, "No."

It was the first time in my life that anyone had allowed me that freedom in writing. Ideas and solutions came to me so fast that I could hardly write them down. I had the time of my life. The counselor pointed out that until my vocabulary increased I would find it frustrating. My ability to express my thoughts in words was so limited.

My mother had remarried, Commander Thomas Dugan, U.S. Navy, during my last year at Shipley. He was on duty in the Pacific. Mother had been a widow and a single parent for nine years.

She asked me what I wanted for a graduation present.

I said, "I want to go back to Coronado. I want to see my friends. Take me to where the boys are!"

I had had enough of girls' schools. I hadn't had a real date since the ones with Bill Eggbeer in Franklin two years earlier.

Mother and I drove the car back to California, with two dogs. My brother and sisters followed later by bus because their schools had gotten out later than mine. The trip was fun, and it was one of the few times I ever spent alone with Mother.

My brother, like me, had had a difficult time at school (undiagnosed dyslexia). He went on to graduate as head boy. He was an excellent tennis player. He loved business and attended Wharton Business School after he graduated from the University of Virginia. My sister Edythe later graduated from Vassar, and my sister Kiki from George Washington University. It was not thought as important that I go on to college because my grades were so poor.

Mother and I arrived in Coronado in the middle of June. I looked up my friends from grade school. I was delighted to see so many of them again. The summer before the war, we had all been sophomores, and it was one of the happiest times I could remember.

I think Mother was worried that I would become romantically involved with one of my male classmates, but all I wanted to do was have a good time, go swimming, dancing, and to the movies, and just talk. I wanted to feel freedom and try to catch up with a part of my life that I had missed.

One day, while backing the car out of the garage, I knocked down one of the wooden garage doors. It fell into the street. I was terrified that Mother might find out and stop me from driving. I stopped the car, got out, and picked up the wooden door and balanced it against the garage and fence. That night I had a date with a young navy ensign. I told him about the door. He said, "It's impossible. You couldn't have lifted that door by yourself."

I wanted to prove to him that I could. So we walked to the door. I couldn't move it! We spent some time that night talking about adrenalin release under stress. I had moved that door because of fear, which had released the adrenalin into my system that had given me that additional strength. This was possibly my first intellectual discussion.

By the end of summer I had to make up my mind whether I wanted to go to work at a dress shop or to go to college. College won, hands down! I enrolled at San Diego State. I commuted between Coronado and San Diego every morning, getting up at five-thirty in order to make the eight o'clock class. I chose trigonometry, and my stepfather suggested accounting.

He said, "It would be a good course for a woman to take."

My counselor suggested a sociology course which she taught, Marriage and the Family; I received an A in her course. It was so easy; it was common sense. My mother had been married three times, divorced once, and widowed once. I knew the difference between a good husband and a bad one.

One day our teacher passed around slips of paper, each with different topics on them. We were to give a ten-minute lecture on the topic we drew. My topic was "The By-products of Illegal Sex Expression." I researched my subject, and lecturing about it was fun.

The next summer Jane and Phyllis Murray came out to spend the summer with my family.

During the afternoons, the three of us taught dancing to the sailors at the United Service Organization. Then we went out with the officers at night. Some of them were ninety-day wonders (men who enlisted in the navy and, after attending college training for ninety days, received commissions as junior grade officers).

Because of the tremendous influx of young officers into San Diego, an admiral's wife started a new club. It was specifically set up so that the young men could meet carefully chosen young women.

The Murray twins, my sister Kiki, two other friends, and I went to the first dance. It was a little awkward at first, but soon we were all dancing. There were many more men than women. While we were dancing, an announcement was made over the loudspeaker, "Will all the girls come to the ladies' room. A coat is missing."

I joked with my dancing partner, George Fleming, "They've caught me!"

He said, "I'll wait for you."

The coat was found, and when I went back, there was George waiting for me. We danced the rest of the night together. The next night my brother was having a beach party, and I needed someone to help me chaperone. I asked George if he would like to help me out. He did, and from then on he was a fixture around the house. He loved to cook and my mother thought that was grand.

My stepfather returned from the Pacific that summer. The war was still going on. The boys I had known in school were now all shipped overseas, and one was in a concentration camp in Germany.

George was stationed at the Navy Amphibious Base. He was to be transferred overseas as soon as he finished his training. We were going steady by the end of the summer, and we decided to be married in September. I did not go back to college. George told me later that he was impressed with me partly because my father was a captain, and because he liked my large family. George was an only child. As for myself, I was quite sure that no one else would ask me to marry.

# CHAPTER 5

## MARRIAGE/MIRAGE

George and I were married at Christ Church, Coronado, where I had been baptized and confirmed. Jane, Kiki, and Edythe were my bridesmaids.

My parents found a little house near town for us to buy. It needed a lot of repair; but they helped us with the down payment, and we rented half of it. It was hard work fixing it up, but we enjoyed doing it. Buying houses and doing them over, then selling them, was to become a way of life for us. We had car payments, house payments, and very little money left over. We were always planning for the future. For fun we used to buy the Sunday funnies on Saturday night. We were so young. I was eighteen and he was twenty when we were married. We felt very secure with each other. And although we used to kid each other, "If we don't get along we will get a divorce," we never meant it.

When the war ended in August of 1945, George decided to return to college on the G.I. bill. We packed the car with our treasures and motored east. It was hot.

We lived in Boston during the winters of those years while George was in college, and we stayed with my family in Jamestown during the summers. On January 25, 1947, our daughter Elizabeth was born. I was twenty-one.

In Boston we found a large basement apartment. It was rent-free, but I had to do the laundry for the family (with five children) that owned the house. It was a full-time job for me, particularly the ironing. George's job was to take out the trash.

When George graduated, he had many offers of work. He decided to take the job that paid the most, $225 a month, working for a chemical company at Marcus Hook, Pennsylvania.

We found a dear old eighteenth century farmhouse outside Philadelphia. It was terribly run-down, but we bought it. I became pregnant with our second child, Thomas, and got a hideous case of poison ivy. Living on a farm taught me one thing—I would never want to retire to the country. I want to be near a drugstore and a movie house.

Mother found George another job that paid more, in Baltimore, Maryland. If all went well, there was a chance he might end up as manager of an automobile dealership. He took the job. I stayed on the farm. I was by then seven months pregnant and we thought it best that I stay where my obstetrician was. Two weeks after Thomas was born, in November, 1948, the children and I moved to Baltimore.

But when the automobile dealership changed hands, George was fired, through no fault of his own. It was quite a blow. I returned to Jamestown with the children while he hunted for another job. In three months he found one in Providence, Rhode Island.

We stayed in Jamestown and we had a happy time that year. The children were by then two and four. Our house was on a hill, and from the windows we could see Narragansett Bay. At night we could see the lights of the navy ships as they sailed up the bay. We had many friends. One of our closest was Allison Bunkley. It was his mother who had originally told my mother about the island. George and I named Allison to be little Liz's godfather. He was a professor of Hispanic studies at Princeton University. He was my age, twenty-five.

Allison asked me one day, "Why didn't you finish college?"

"I was too dumb," I answered.

He said nothing, but came to see me the next day, with a book under his arm.

I told him the story of how my mother had told George, just before we were married, "Remember, George, Elizabeth is not bright enough to come in out of the rain." Mother, George, and I had all laughed.

Allison said, "That was not funny, Elizabeth. And you are not dumb."

I asked him, "How do you know?"

He said, "I have listened to you talk. You know a great deal about a lot of subjects. You also have a lot of common sense, and nothing is common about common sense! A great many people have none at all. You particularly know a great deal more about religion than most people. I have brought you this book about the history and thought of early Hebrew people, when they were nomads. Read it, and I will discuss it with you as you go along."

I learned years later that Allison had given brother Lionel a similar talk, assuring him that he was not dumb. It was Allison who was responsible for Lionel's being sent to Storm-King School. Allison had gone there as a young boy, and it was there that Allison's genius had been discovered and nurtured.

During the years when George and I were moving around, it was always reassuring to get back to Jamestown every summer, if only for a short two-week vacation.

George was transferred to Lancaster, Pennsylvania, where, in November, 1950, our third child, Ellanor (Ellie), was born. Those next years, with three children under the age of six, were the hardest years of my life.

In Lancaster we rented a house. I did all the family laundry by hand. We had no washing machine or wringer. The winters were bitterly cold and icy. George and I were of the old school. The husband must always be emotionally supported. It was accepted that the wife could get blamed for anything that went wrong. I was supposed to be a superwoman, wife and mother. And yet the jobs I performed were always considered menial—taking care of the children and the house, cooking, laundry, whatever. I didn't fight back. I didn't know any better. I was emotionally and physically exhausted. To this day, I never pass a woman with dark, deep circles under her eyes and little children without tears coming to my eyes.

After two years in Lancaster, George had an opportunity to work for Koppers Company in Pittsburgh, Pennsylvania. He took the job. We moved to Sewickley, Pennsylvania, and rented an apartment. A year passed before we found a house to buy, 29 Beaver Street. It was a large Victorian house near town, with eleven rooms, all in disrepair. I loved it and felt that I would be there the rest of my life.

One morning I was sitting at the kitchen table reading the newspaper when I saw a big ad, "This is your last chance to be an Arthur Murray dancing teacher." I telephoned a friend and asked if she would come over and baby-sit with the children while I went down and applied for the job at Arthur Murray's. I knew I had to go. The children where by then seven, five, and three. I had never had time to recuperate from childbearing. We had moved twenty-one times since our marriage nine years before. I was someone's wife, daughter, sister, mother, but who was *I*? Even my husband didn't know. The night before, we had gone out to dinner with an older couple from the office. I had talked about myself.

The hostess had said, "Your life sounds fascinating. Tell me about it."

When I realized that she was sincere, I was flattered and started to tell her my story, beginning with being born at Walter Reed Hospital in Washington, D.C.

George interrupted, saying that he wanted to tell the story. "She was born in Franklin, Pennsylvania, an only child. Her cousin was Woodrow Wilson."

I had been horrified. He was telling of my mother's life, not mine—and he hadn't even noticed the difference!

I did go to Arthur Murray's and I did get the job. I taught dancing for six happy months. I knew I was a teacher and my name was Elizabeth.

The next year we renovated the house. The children had their own bedrooms. The kitchen was done over, with a washer and dryer. The living room was lovely. The dining room had been the old music room and had corner columns and small crystal chandeliers. At last we were all at home, and I was very happy. George was delighted with his job. Those earlier years of struggle had paid off. We were settled in our new home and living the life we had prepared for all those years.

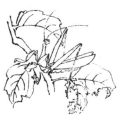

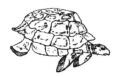

## CHAPTER 6

## PSYCHIATRIC EVALUATION

*The more faithfully you listen to
the voice within you, the better
you will hear what is sounding
outside.*
...Dag Hammarskjold
*Markings*

My mother had been a great believer in psychiatric evaluations ever since she had started seeing Dr. Nar because of problems she and my stepfather were having following his retirement from the navy. Dr. Nar was an outstanding psychiatrist and neurologist. He practiced in Washington, D.C.

Mother wanted all of her children to see him, for she didn't feel that we were leading our lives as well as we might. I was happy living in Sewickley and had a lovely husband and three healthy children; but I went down to Washington to see Dr. Nar.

After the hour was up he said, "I find you in good health, Mrs. Fleming, with only three things to suggest you might want to work on or improve on. One, you have some trouble expressing your feelings. Two, you have trouble expressing what you are thinking. Three, you have trouble formulating what you want."

I was amazed! He had pointed out the three things that I had become aware of and had started working on myself.

I asked him, "Is this something you can help me with?"

He answered, "Yes."

"How long would it take?" I replied.

He said, "About fifteen hours."

So my schedule was set. For four months I went to Washington by bus every other week for an appointment. I had a two-hour session and then returned to Sewickley. The bus took six hours each way, but I found that very beneficial. It gave me time to think things over—on the way down, what I wanted to say, and on the way home, what Dr. Nar had talked about.

The first thing he asked me was to tell him the story of my life as a child. I spoke of the second grade experience when my teacher had made me change my writing hand from left to right. Through treatment, it became clear that the changing of my writing hand had closed off my early emotions from my conscious memory.

For the use of my right hand I had used my left brain. Earlier, when I had used my left hand, I had used my right brain. Movement of each side of the human body is controlled by the opposite side of the brain.

By the end of the fifteen hours I was fully aware of using both sides of my brain, and I had reexperienced my early childhood feelings.

We discovered that my early years were a time of intense emotion. In 1932, when I was six, my father was given command of the United States Navy ship *Ganett*. It was a small ship with a hand-picked crew. Their assignment was to survey and map the Aleutian Islands. They were gone for six months. It was the longest and loneliest period of my life. My father was one of the few people to whom I could talk, and he would listen to me. I loved him very much. I had no adult to talk to while he was gone. Mother was ill and very despondent at being pregnant again. She scolded me when I did something bad. So I was very, very good. I wanted my daddy to come home.

After my father returned, the family took a three-month trip to Europe. My parents were trying to work out problems they had. We children were put in a boarding school in Brussels during that time. I still remember playing with the other children there. None of us spoke the same language, and yet we were able to talk to each other. When the radio was on, I could understand all the words to the French songs.

We returned to Coronado. Mother and Father had decided to get a divorce. Father took us children aside and told us, "Your mother and I are going to be divorced. I will be leaving. I want you all to be good. Elizabeth, you are the oldest, and I want you to help your mother with the younger children, your brother and sisters. Lionel, you are the man of the family. I expect you to behave as such and help your sisters." Ever since, my brother and I have been able to discuss serious subjects together.

Mother remarried. Her new husband was Gill Goetz, an army aviator. Tragically, he died from a sudden illness only thirteen days after their marriage.

Mother used to cry a lot. Sometimes she would be in terrible pain and scream, falling to the floor and writhing. (It was later diagnosed as gallbladder attacks.) My sister Kiki would come and get me, saying, "Mother's sick again." Or, "Mother's crying again. Come and do something." I took it very seriously and would go in and try to help and comfort her.

I can still hear Dr. Nar asking, "How did you feel about that, Elizabeth?"

No one had ever asked me how I *felt* before. I had been asked what I thought, but never what I felt. During those discussions with Dr. Nar, I was able to open those memories and feelings. I was able to integrate both sides of my brain. God, it was exciting to feel my full energy.

Through therapy I found out that the people I felt had accepted and loved me, just the way I was, were my father, Bill Goetz (my first stepfather), and Allison Bunkley. My mother and George, I felt, accepted me with strings attached. I would love you, but you haven't done this or that. I would love you if you did this or that (lose weight, work harder, keep the house cleaner, wash the car, help me more...). I used to call that, "I'd love you *if*," "I'd love you *but*." Bless their hearts, they were trying to make me perfect in their own eyes.

Dr. Nar discussed and explained the concepts of "roles" and "patterns," pointing out and illustrating where they occurred in my own life. Until then I thought roles were something you ate, and patterns were something you followed when you cut out dress material.

A pattern that showed up in my life was similar to one that affected my mother during her childhood. She had been a beautiful child but had always been told how ugly she was. She did not say the same to me. She knew how badly that had hurt her. But the ambivalent emotional messages (love and hate) that she received from her mother she passed down to me by saying it was all right that I was stupid.

When this pattern was brought to my attention, I looked at Dr. Nar and said, "If my grandmother did that to my mother, and she in turn subconsciously did it to me, am I doing the same to my daughter little Liz?"

Dr. Nar said, "Yes."

I could hardly wait to get home. There sat little Liz in the kitchen, having a snack after school. She had already had to repeat the third grade because of her poor reading.

I looked at her and said, "Has anyone ever told you that not only are you beautiful but you are also brilliant?" Her eyes misted over, and she whispered, "No, never."

I could see the pain in her little face and I thought how marvelous it was that I had been made aware of a negative family pattern and given the opportunity to apologize, particularly to someone so young.

A role that I often played by not speaking up for myself was that of martyr. As soon as I began asserting myself and speaking up, that passed. By my last visit to Washington, Dr. Nar had helped me to express my anger and not to be afraid of it any longer. It was a new experience. I had never been able to verbalize anger before. When I was a child I was not even supposed to *hate* spinach.

On my last visit to Dr. Nar I said, "I have known a little sorrow and therefore have a little compassion. But you have known so much sorrow and have so much compassion."

That was a very happy time for me. The clouds had lifted. George liked his work. Best of all, the children were older (nine, seven, and five) and all in school. The house was easy to keep in order, and we had a new kitchen. A cleaning lady came in to help me once a week. I realized that by the time I was forty I would be "free." The children would be grown, and I would have time for myself.

Once my mother came to visit us. She asked me if I wanted to go to Europe with her. I just laughed and said, "Everything is going so well here. I can't leave my husband and the children for three months." But George would have agreed to it, if I had wanted to go.

At about that time, George's mother retired. She wanted to come and live with us for a while, until she got settled. George didn't want her to come, but I said, "We can't just leave her."

I referred to the good Samaritan. "You can't just leave them on the road, George."

Not until later did I realize that the sermon I had heard on the good Samaritan had not been given correctly. It was important that the traveler had stopped and helped the sick man, but even more important that he had taken the sick man to an inn, not to his own home.

At first I thought the visit was working out. She was delighted to take care of the children, which gave George and me more freedom. We made a little efficiency apartment for her in the back wing of the house. I enjoyed listening to her talk about her childhood, and she seemed fond of me. She became part of our life. Then something went wrong. She was hurt whenever anyone came over to the house and she was not included. She began to complain to George about the way I was bringing up the children. It was time for her to find an apartment of her own, but she was in no hurry to go gracefully, even when we found suitable places for her. It became quite awkward.

I went to see Dr. Nar in Washington and talked to him about the problem of resettling my mother-in-law. By taking her into our house when she did not have one of her own, I had set up an environment for jealousy. The doctor carefully pointed out that it was not my place to ask her to leave. George must do it. She was *his* mother.

When I got back from Washington I didn't feel well and decided to see the doctor. He told me I was pregnant. There went my plans for being free of the responsibilities of children by the time I was forty. After talking it over with George, I telephoned my mother and asked, "May I please change my mind and take you up on that trip to Europe? I'm pregnant again."

Soon, there I was, three months pregnant, sitting down to my first breakfast aboard a ship of the Holland America Lines. Mother and I had been placed at a table with four other people. They were all my age, twenty-nine. There were two war brides returning to see their families in Holland, one Dutch Air Corps pilot, and Jack Lauritzen, who was to become a close friend. He had just received his doctorate in nuclear physics from Cal Tech. He was taking a four-month sabbatical before returning to Washington, D.C., to work for the National Bureau of Standards. I had lots of fun talking with him and listening to him talk about physics. He had worked at Los Alamos, New Mexico, where the first cyclotron had been built.

Mother and I had a grand trip. I saw England, France, and Spain. We were in Spain nearly two months, visiting friends. I returned after three months, having had a great rest. The children were in marvelous shape, and all seemed about the same at 29 Beaver Street.

My mother-in-law soon found an apartment in town.

George and I had our first serious talk about our marriage and what we wanted and expected. We decided that ours was a good marriage and worth working on.

Our son George was born in 1965, a delightful redhaired boy. Those were agreeable years. I was growing up, and so was our family. We had close friends and led a pleasant social life. We had joined a country club just a few blocks away from the house. I took the children swimming every day during the summers. George was on the vestry at church, and our family went every Sunday. We were very fond of the minister. The first three years after little George was born were a loving and special time.

But something happened to change that when I found out that I was pregnant for the fifth time. The pressure became too great for George.

He told my brother, "I don't think I can go through with it."

George was right. He couldn't go through with it. When I was three months pregnant, he told me he was in love with someone else, but didn't know whether or not he wanted a divorce so as to be able to marry her.

We both went to see Dr. Nar in Washington. Our marriage indeed was in its greatest crisis. If I could remain supportive during this period, George might come out of it and be able to work through his ambivalence toward women.

I did hold on for a long time, with the help of my obstetrician, Dr. Pink, who was very familiar with the vocabulary and problems of psychiatric evaluation, having been through psychoanalysis himself. But George was going out nearly every night. When I asked him what I was to do if the baby came while he was away, he gave me ten dollars and told me to call a cab.

I knew that I needed more psychiatric help when one night in the living room I felt as though George and the girl he was seeing were coming down the hall to kill me. I had had enough psychiatric background to realize that it was I who was so angry at those two that I could have killed them. I was determined that nothing would upset my pregnancy. Dr. Nar, in Washington, was too far away. So I called a psychiatrist in Pittsburgh and asked if he would see me.

The house outwardly went on the same. Liz was in private day school, where she had gone after repeating the third grade. Tommy and Ellie were in public school, and little George was just three years old and at home.

I started to read because of my need for company. I found a book left by the former tenants, *Four Famous Greek Plays*. I read *Oedipus the King*, by Sophocles, and *Medea*, by Euripides. I was fascinated by *Oedipus*, and constantly aware of Sigmund Freud's use of the material in his work. When I read *Medea*, I could not understand why Freud had not taken that work as seriously. I told my doctor so.

I would talk to the psychiatrist, who was by now our marriage counselor, much the way I had to Dr. Nar, about things that I was thinking about, concepts that I was working with, whatever came into my mind. I knew the game with George was a waiting one and that the calmer I could be about it, the better. There was still a chance that, if I didn't bungle it, turn George away, he might decide to come back to me.

The last two months before the baby was born were not easy, but they did pass. The baby was born in November, 1959. I named him John Richard Lionel. John, for gift of God; Richard, for Richard the Lion-Hearted; and Lionel, after my brother. I felt that the new baby had survived the turmoil during the pregnancy and he deserved a fitting name.

Soon after the baby was born, I decided my marriage was over. Although George said he hadn't made up his mind, he was still seeing the other woman. I could wait no longer. I wanted a divorce.

I told my close friend Ann what I was going to do. "Tonight, when George goes out, I'm going to go up on the porch and throw his bed over the rail. When he sees it, when he comes home, I'm going to tell him to *shape up or ship out*." I could make another life for myself, without being married to George. And my friend thought the idea of pitching the bed out was a grand one. So that night I did it. George was totally amazed! He asked me please to wait and let him phone the psychiatrist, our marriage counselor.

I said, "But it's too late at night to call."

He said, "No, it's not. The doctor said I could call him any time at night." When George got back from the phone he said, "I got the doctor and he gave us an appointment for tomorrow morning. Will you please go with me?"

I said, "All right. I'll go."

The next morning we were in the doctor's office by ten. He asked to see George first, and then me. I told the doctor about throwing the bed off the porch, and telling George to "shape up or ship out." Furthermore, I told him, I wanted a divorce because I was tired of waiting for George to make up his mind as to which woman he wanted for wife and lover.

The doctor asked me, "Is there anything that would bother you about getting a divorce?"

I said, "Yes. I don't know what I will do with my sexual energy."

He listened unemotionally and then said, "I think you ought to sign yourself into a psychiatric hospital."

I thought he was joking and started to laugh. "You're kidding," I said.

He answered, "On the contrary, Mrs. Fleming. I am very serious."

"But why?" I asked.

He answered, "I feel you have been under an enormous emotional stress and that you should go to the hospital and have a complete psychological evaluation."

Oh boy, that did it. Something inside me snapped. *No one* was going to say, insinuate, or imply that I was dumb, stupid, or crazy—ever again.

I was tired of hearing it.

I had had it!

I knew I was a healthy human being—physically and emotionally.

The time I had spent with Dr. Nar had proven it to me.

George had said that, if we got a divorce, I could go back to dancing and he would take the children. But the children were *not* going to be taken away from me. I wasn't afraid to be tested by anyone. If, to prove once and for all that I was sane, I had to sign myself into a psychiatric hospital—I'd do it.

The doctor suggested that I postpone filing for divorce until after the hospital testing. Before leaving his office, I turned to him and asked, "How long will I have to stay in the hospital?" He answered, "The shortest time would be two weeks, the longest, two years."

I thought to myself, "I'll be out in two weeks."

I signed myself into the hospital on the day after Christmas. It was five weeks before I was released, with a clean bill of health. But, at last, I had the psychiatric hospital papers to prove that I was in good emotional and physical health.

However, it was to take many years for me to get over the trauma of being hospitalized and of being isolated from my children—except for their half-hour visits once a week.

Dr. Pink, my obstetrician, who had seen me while I was in the psychiatric hospital, later said, "You might have been neurotic at that time, but you were never psychotic." When I asked my hospital psychiatrist what had been wrong with me, she told me I had had a gross inferiority complex.

Two months after my release from the hospital, I was walking across a street in Pittsburgh when I saw a man who had only one arm. He was crossing the street, coming toward me. Eight years later I wrote a poem about it. The memory of that moment had stayed clearly in my mind.

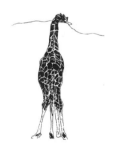

### I Saw a Man a Year Ago

*I saw a man a year ago,*
*or was it eight or eighty?*
*He had no arm. I had no heart...*
*Yet, when our eyes beheld each other*
*across the intersection (that sea of*
*humans scattered yet controlled by*
*blinking lights)*
*we recognized each other.*
*He saw my heart...*
*I saw his arm...*
*We did not speak*
*across the sea but,*
*I saw him and he saw me*
                              *and*
*in that whole moment of eternity*
*I was received and so was he.*

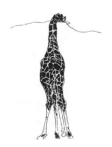

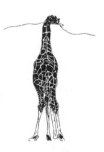

# CHAPTER 7

## CREATIVITY AND HEALTH

*Life only demands from you the strength*
*you possess. Only one feat is possible—*
*not to have run away.*
. . . Dag Hammarskjold
*Markings*

Time passed slowly at first. I took it day-by-day or, sometimes, moment-by-moment. Painting and reading were my outlets. I was at home alone with little children. Only the oldest three were in school. I didn't own a car; but our house was only three blocks from the village, and we could walk to the store, movies, and church.

At first, I met a few people in town who would greet me with nervous smiles, and in condescending voices ask me, "How are you feeling, Elizabeth?"

"Just fine, thank you," I would respond.

But this question used to irritate me. It was none of their business how I felt. I finally decided that I was going to answer the next person that asked me that personal question, just to startle them, "As depressed as hell! How do you feel?"

I thought that was a better answer than, "I feel with my hands. How do you feel?"

I chuckled to myself over these imaginary answers of mine; I never used them. Once I had them, no one ever asked me the question in public again.

Viktor Frankl wrote in his book, *Man's Search for Meaning*, "No explanations are needed for those who have been inside, and the others will understand neither how we felt then nor how we feel now."

Doctor Frankl is a psychiatrist who wrote of his experiences as a prisoner of war in a German camp. This was the group I had identified with while I was in the hospital. He wrote of his own "inborn optimism." Also, he spoke of the "grim sense of humor" some of the prisoners of war used. Humor, he said, was "one of the soul's weapons" in the fight for self-preservation.

He spoke of the bitterness that some prisoners experienced after being released and returning home. When I read that part, I remembered my own feeling of bitterness in the hospital.

One day I had knelt by my hospital bed and prayed, "Dear God, please make me angry, not bitter." In time, I knew I could work through anger, but even then I realized I would not be able to handle the negative emotions of bitterness or spite. I knew I would need all the positive energy I could find.

For me, the most penetrating lines in *Man's Search for Meaning* were, "The crowning experience of all, for the homecoming man, is the wonderful feeling that, after all he has suffered, there is nothing he need fear any more—except his God."

George made child support payments, which were enough to pay the mortgage and utility bills each month. My stepfather sent me a check every week to pay for the groceries. But my mother was worried about my long-term financial situation, for I received no alimony. She found long-term real estate investments in California for me.

The houses in California were financed through six thousand dollars my mother gave me and two or sometimes three mortgages that were placed in my name on each house. It was nip and tuck those early years—but it worked! I could stay at home and take care of the children. That was what I wanted to do. My time and energy would be put into the raising of my children. I never regretted that decision. I am so thankful that I was able to have the choice.

I found three statements to be worth their weight in gold.

I used the first one when someone tried to put a label on me or something I believed in. If I thought their statement was unacceptable, I said, *"You said that, not I!"*

I used the second when someone suggested something I did not want to be part of. I said, *"That is your problem, not mine!"*

The third statement was, *"Do not move until you have a reason for moving."* If you do, you take your problems with you. Work your problems out where you are, and then you are free—to move for a reason.

By the time I returned home from the hospital, God was my friend and my companion. Yet I remember becoming wildly angry with Him and calling out, "I hate you God!"

He answered back, "So what else is new?"

He had accepted my anger, and I was no longer afraid. He had answered me back once at the hospital. Before going to sleep one night I was saying my prayers over and over and He just told me, "You are tired, go to sleep!"

Those first few months at home were like being in a new place, a new psychological and spiritual dimension. I was still raw and felt like a leper, an untouchable. My life seemed fragmented. Growth, confrontation, and solitude were never smooth sailing, at least not for me.

I remember looking at myself in the mirror when I returned home from the hospital. The hospital stay plus the new baby, who was only three months old, had left me looking like an invalid. As a child, body surfing and dancing had helped to give me good physical balance and health. I wanted to get back to that feeling again.

I had read an article in *The New York Times* about exercising. The theory was that one should go through the physical motions of a newborn baby and work up to those of a toddler. The instructions were as follows:

1. Curl up on the floor in the fetal position, then stretch out and turn so that you are on your back. Stretch your arms and legs slowly. Move yourself around.

2. Try to turn onto your stomach. Then wiggle like a fish out of water. Inch your way around in a circle.

3. Try to get onto your knees and hands and start crawling—slowly at first, then faster and faster.

4. Then stand up and walk...

It was a ten-minute exercise. There I was the next day, crawling around the floor like a baby.

A widow, shortly after the death of her husband, wrote,"I felt that I had fallen into the bottom of a well, but as long as I was there I decided I might as well start housekeeping." It was good advice. I decided I would do the same. Indeed, to say that I had fallen into the bottom of a well would be putting it mildly. I felt like a discarded piece of old baggage. I felt drained and raw.

Courage moves, and fear hinders. I was afraid that I couldn't handle the responsibility of raising the children by myself. So I decided that they were God's children, not mine. Therefore it was up to Him to take the responsibility for raising them. He had chosen me to be their mother, so it was up to Him to direct me.

One rainy day, I was sitting in a comfortable chair in the living room. I asked myself, "What would I really like to do, if I had no responsibility?"

The answer came, "Sit in this chair."

"How could I do that legitimately—and not feel guilty about it?"

"I could become an intellectual. They don't feel guilty sitting in a chair and reading or contemplating."

"How can I become an intellectual?"

"Start reading."

I'd heard "You can't read!" all through my childhood. As a hereditary dyslexic, taking in words in all their levels of meaning, I was aware that the phrase carried with it a double message. "You can't read!" meant I was unable to read. It also meant I was *not allowed* to read. For me, reading was taboo.

That afternoon a neighbor asked if she could get me anything at the library. I had read in the newspaper that a new book by a psychiatrist named Carl Jung had just been published, and it sounded interesting. I asked her to pick me up a copy. As it turned out, it had a lot of "dirty" information in it. (My definition of "dirty" was anything I wasn't supposed to know about—a hangover from my childhood.)

Marlborough Books ran an ad in the newspaper saying that they would mail any book ordered, in an unmarked envelope. I ordered a book by Jean-Paul Sartre. Somehow it was still important for me to keep it a secret. I didn't want anyone to know that I was ordering a book because they might make fun of me for thinking I wanted to be an intellectual.

Sartre's *Of Human Freedom* arrived by mail in the plain wrapper as promised. I wasn't disappointed. I enjoyed marvelous chapters, like "The Meaning of Existence: Nausea"; "Freedom to Create: The Psychology of Imagination"; "Freedom to Have, to Do, to Be: Being and Nothingness"; and "Freedom from Persecution."

I read lines like "The world of explanations and reasons is not the world of existence," and "...to play with the absurdity of the world," and "To exist is simply to be there; those who exist let themselves be encountered...."

I was now thirty-two and asking questions: Who am I? Why am I feeling different from everybody else? What does my life stand for? Nobody else I knew was doing this. That is why I turned to books for some kind of comfort, understanding, reassurance, and information. The right books sometimes seemed to fall into my hands; for example *Human Destiny*, by Lecomte du Nouy and *Pain, Sex and Time*, by Gerald Heard. Both authors reassured me that some people are just born different from others. There you are, with a different perspective on life. You are different from anyone else you know, and it's all right.

I started educating myself, through reading. If any word or concept caught my fancy, I went to the library and took out all the books I could find on the subject. Once, the word *psychic* captured my imagination. There weren't many books that had that word in the title twenty years ago. The two I found were Jung's *Psyche and Symbol* and a paperback whose title I have forgotten. It was the biography of a psychic woman who had lived in New York. Because of my dyslexia, one book was no harder for me to read than the other, and I was always glad that I had gotten the broader picture by reading both books.

When I was lonely, and when I was trying to make sense out of human love and friendship, it was through Miguel De Unamuno's *Tragic Sense of Life* and Martin Buber's *I and Thou* that I received understanding. Buber said of love, "Through the graciousness of its comings and the solemn sadness of its goings it leads you away to the Thou in which the parallel lines of relations meet. It does not help to sustain you in life, it only helps you to glimpse eternity."

My dear teacher and friend Allison Bunkley had been killed in an accident when he was only twenty-six. It was a delight to be reading the books about existentialism of which he had so often spoken. Unamuno, the Spanish philosopher, had been one of his favorites. I went through these books like a kid in a candy box. The one advantage of my being so ignorant in the fields of philosophy and theology was that there was so much to learn.

Unamuno spoke of friendships. "...a new friend enriches our spirit, not so much by what he gives us of himself, as by what he causes us to discover in our own selves, something which, if we had never known him, would have lain in us undeveloped...."

While reading, I never looked up a word I didn't know in the dictionary until the author used it for the third time. If he used a word three times, I felt it must be an important part of his vocabulary. I looked it up—and I learned it. Certain authors who are considered difficult are not. It's just that each author has his own vocabulary and uses certain words that are not in the reader's vocabulary.

The theologian Paul Tillich, for example, uses the word *ontological*. After looking it up in a number of dictionaries, I found that *ontology* means "a science or study of being." Every time I came across the word in his writing I would just say to myself, "Think big, Elizabeth." I knew he would not be discussing something trivial.

If I go on about books and authors, it's because they were my teachers during the eight years of my self-education following my stay in the hospital. It was a period of catching-up to my peers and the current thoughts of the day. The companionship of thoughts and concepts was mine through reading. I could no longer afford the poverty of ignorance.

All the adjectives and prepositions in novels clouded up the meaning for me, for my mind processed each word individually. That's why I read books on philosophy and psychiatry and theology. My mind was like a race horse raring to go. There was so much to know. It was as though some chain had been holding me back before. The chain of ridicule is sometimes the strongest.

Just before Christmas I took a course at church in how to make Christmas decorations and ornaments. The teacher taught us to use what we could find around the yard—pine cones, nuts, and interesting pieces of wood. It was a marvelous feeling to create something that had never been seen before, to make something out of nothing.

One day, after the four-week course was over, I felt a tremendous inner surge of creative energy. I went outdoors and slowly walked around the house. I was trying to find something to work with—to create with. No acorns, no nuts, nothing. So I returned to the house and went down to the basement, in desperation to find something to work with. There it was: house paints, brushes, and old building panels made of beaverboard.

I started to paint that night.

The hours from eleven-thirty in the evening to two in the morning were mine. The children were in bed and the baby was fed. The house was quiet. The night was still. Down to the basement I would go. There, undisturbed, I could let my feelings express themselves. I told an artist I knew, what I was doing.

She said, "Get those paintings out of the basement and put them on the living room mantel."

She gave me only two pieces of advice: "The wrong color? Let the canvas alone for twenty-four hours. It might turn out to be the best color you ever mixed." And "Use the same color in three places or more, in case you can't mix the same color again."

The assistant minister visited one day and, seeing the paintings on the wall, said, "Not everyone hangs their psyche all over their living room walls."

My nicest compliment came from my older daughter, Elizabeth. She was doing the grocery shopping, and I had told her that she couldn't buy any treats for the children. Upon returning home from the store, she saw my latest painting, *A Time To Be Born*. My style had changed and she thought I had bought the painting. She gave me hell for having spent so much money. Flattery was not what I painted for. I painted because I had to. But it was great to get such positive feedback.

I was finding that, to have a truly balanced life, I had to have creative outlets. Writing, painting, and music are the three given by the well-known psychiatrist and author Karl Menninger. I was not musical. That left writing and painting. Painting was natural for me. The energy within me from the new concepts I was learning about while reading was screaming to be expressed. There was no person I knew who was interested in what I was discovering and comprehending. Often, when trying to strike up a conversation about one of the authors or books, I would get the reply, "Oh yes, I had to read that in college years ago."

Maybe, if I had been better with words, I would have turned to writing then. But I had been indoctrinated too well, "If you can't spell you can't write."

I received a lot of support through reading Benedetto Croce. He says to create because you must or just want to. It has nothing to do with whether you are a good or a bad artist. Create because it is a part of you, an expression of you. It is for fun. It is an outlet for creative energy that, if not given expression, turns in against the self.

When that strange feeling would come over me, that intangible feeling of energy within, I would sometimes take a blank sheet of paper and a pencil, sit down, and start writing.

How long ago, I held your hand.
How long ago, I wept.
How long ago, you went away and I alone did stay.

Sometimes I would ask a question and let the answer come. Sometimes I would write a petition.

Dear God, as the originator of my being, may I ask you where now to turn in this finite world? In this finite life of mine, somewhere things have gone astray, or perhaps they never were headed in the right direction. Have I fallen in love with people who are incapable of feeling love? Is it an early childhood pattern that I am carrying on as an adult? If this is so, and so it seems to be, where do I go from here? The answer: You do not go anywhere, but turn around to Me and start anew.

Who will give me the strength to start this search anew? The answer: It will not be a search as you know it, but a walk through beauty, repose, joy, truth, companionship, and love.

Shall I once again marry? The answer: This is no time to answer a question like that. It has so little to do with life and living anyway, if you could only realize this.

What shall I live for? The answer: Why must you have something to live for? The truth is to live each day, each moment, that I, your God, have given you, on this finite planet where you find yourself today. Say hello to life. Enjoy it, for you may be here but for a short time. Treat each day as though it were your last, and you will find your days filled with wonders and love and light.

The question, Did the answers come from within myself or from God? is trivial. "The kingdom of heaven is within."

George Washington Carver said it best, "The artist—his writings, his weaving, his music, his painting—are just expressions of his soul in search of Truth."

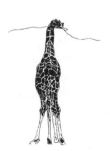

# CHAPTER 8

## RE-ENTRY: Reassurance and Night School

Emotional reassurance was something I now had to find for myself, anyplace I could find it—horoscopes in the newspaper, blank verse writing, talking to God, reading. It wasn't that I had to believe it. It was just reassuring to get some kind of "feedback" when I was living alone with little children.

This is a poem I wrote one morning—as though my old teacher Allison were talking to me:

To Elizabeth

Your life will change.
Be not afraid.
"This is the last
For which
The first was made."

I also wrote on that morning

Pierce through the foul smell of lies
Pierce through the dimming of our senses
Walk through the darkness
to the other side.
Burst forth to life.
I am not caught in a corner
of a universe.
But am a pulsing part of it.

And then, quieting down,

Love is forever the growing force of God.
Birth and death are just statements of time.
Love is the messenger of eternity.

I had found Kierkegaard's definition of Christian courage: "The courage to stand alone, in fear and trembling, before one's God and take this awesome responsibility unto oneself." When I wanted to talk about these concepts, no one else wanted to talk about them; indeed they seemed to frighten people. That was the reason my painting was so satisfactory to me. People will share their thoughts about paintings.

I reevaluated so much during this period. Through Carl Jung's interpretation of *self* I found personal insight: If I wanted to help myself grow, I would have to control my ego, my "I," so that my larger inner self could grow. Sometimes, my "I" would want to do something so badly—like run away from all this responsibility of raising five children by myself. My "I" screamed to say, "Yes!" But, for my total well being, my larger self, it was imperative that I say no.

Where was I going to get this strength?

It would come from the moment during Holy Communion, when the priest would pass me the bread and wine, repeating these words of Jesus, "Take, eat, this is my body, which is given for you." Through the taking of the symbols of bread and wine, I could experience that moment of union with the infinite energy and strength of Jesus.

During my search for more insights and for meaning for my life, I realized that the word *Love* could be inserted in place of the word *Jesus*. This brought a new understanding. Here is an example.

Love suffered and was buried:
And the third day Love rose again
And ascended into heaven,
And sitteth on the right hand of the Father:
And Love shall come again, with glory,
to judge both the quick and the dead;
Whose kingdom shall have no end.

I kept on trying to learn, search, and grow. I was still an Episcopalian—not because I had born into it, but because I enjoyed the service and the fellowship. Also I loved the Christian church as an organization. I felt it had tried to keep the concept of Love alive, and to pass it down through the generations.

I remember my first Christmas alone with the children. I couldn't see how I would be able to face it. Then somewhere I read in an article that if you can't carry on your old traditions, make up some new ones, like serving champagne. I liked that idea. That first Christmas, my daughter Elizabeth stayed up late as Santa's helper, and the last thing she and I did after decorating the tree was to put a bottle of champagne in the icebox for Christmas morning. Champagne for Christmas is now a family tradition for all of us.

Because I was lonely for adult company, I started a "Tuesday Night Club" for singles. There were only three of us: the girl next door, the new assistant minister, and me. Our ages ranged from twenty-one to thirty-two. Each Tuesday night we met at my house at six-thirty. Then all of us would drive in one car to a restaurant. It was usually the same restaurant, an Armenian one just fifteen minutes out of town. The food was good, and the price was right. We each paid for our own dinner.

We had a rule that we would not date each other, but would meet and discuss over dinner our love life or lack of it, or any other subject we wanted. No conversation held was to be repeated outside the group.

For example, I might tell about a dream I had had during the week and the others would listen. When finished, I would say what I thought the dream meant. They might then point out something I had missed, asking, "Why did you skip over that one, Elizabeth?" We would laugh, and then I would have to figure out why I had forgotten or overlooked some important point in my dream.

Our trio provided marvelous emotional support and good company for each of us. Also, it was just plain fun.

I began to think about more formal education after I read this story:

A man wanted to go to college. In talking to a college counselor he said, "I can only go to night school. How long do you think it will take me to receive my degree?"

The counselor answered, "About ten years."

The man said, "That would be much too long! I'll be so old when I graduate."

"How old will you be in ten years if you go to college?" asked the counselor.

"I'll be thirty-nine," the man replied.

"How old will you be in ten years if you *don't* go to college?" asked the counselor.

"I'll be thirty-nine anyway!" the man said.

I realized that time would pass whether I chose college or not. I chose college. A course taken here and there for credit would add up over the years. But, I wondered, would I be able to pass the English SAT (Scholastic Aptitude Test)? Was my fear of ridicule still there? Fortunately, I found I could sign up for courses as a night student without taking entrance exams.

I went to Carnegie Tech, in Pittsburgh, and took freshman psychology. I wanted to learn the vocabulary. Later, I took a course in real-estate management and a course in real-estate appraisal at the University of Pittsburgh. Real estate was the family business and I needed to know that vocabulary also.

Five years after the divorce, the children and I made a happy move to an old house that my family owned, in Bethesda, Maryland. My sisters and my brother generously gave their shares of the house to me—it was mine and the bank's. I decided to move because the house was just twenty minutes outside Washington, D.C. I wanted to enlarge my social group and expose myself and the children to a larger, more cosmopolitan setting.

I was lucky, that first year in Washington, to find a congenial group of people. They were theatre buffs. There were two landscape gardeners, and five research scientists who worked across the street from our house, for the National Institutes of Health. We read everything, from Shakespeare to Sartre's *The Flies*. Each week a different person was assigned to find a play and allocate the character parts.

I was also able to continue with college after our move. What drove me to college this time? I couldn't understand the science section of *Time* magazine. I was seeing words like *quarks* and *quasars*.

Also, I had been thinking about life and death. Some said, "Don't worry about it. We all return to dust. There is no life after death." I said to myself, "If we all return to dust, there is no problem. But, if we do not—and there is life after death—there are two things I had better seriously think about: First, living with myself through all eternity. Second, the concept of Heaven and Hell. What would be my idea of a perfect Hell, for *me*?" That was easy. My idea of a perfect Hell would be one in which I would bore myself to death—through all eternity. I decided to do as much as I could to open my mind to new ideas and concepts!

I went back to college, Montgomery College, Rockville, Maryland. I started with a physics course, and that led me back to algebra and then to calculus. It took me a long time to get up enough nerve to take two special courses, Einstein's Theory of Relativity, and Quantum Mechanics for the Nonmathematician. The professor not only had doctorates in physics and philosophy, but also in theology. He was an outstanding teacher, who used humor as a teaching tool. The classes were small with a cross-section of students, from a seventy-eight-year-old woman who had her doctorate in mathematics to two advanced high-school students. Those two students would read Goethe and Proust as I would read comic books—just for fun.

For the class Einstein's Theory of Relativity, I wrote a paper, "Einstein and Dyslexia." By this time four of my children had been diagnosed as having hereditary dyslexia, as had my brother and I. (My daughter Ellie was not diagnosed until she was twenty-nine.)

During the oral presentation of my paper, I brought up the concept of a dyslexic's not using the usual words, *up, down, left,* and *right,* in describing location of a form or object. The dyslexic sees an object placed on a wall or blackboard, without "up," "downs," "tops," or 'bottoms."

Another point I brought up—dyslexics have no trouble in learning Chinese characters because each character represents a concept. Dyslexics love concepts. It's individual words that get them down. I had started a course in Chinese myself that year. I had done so miserably in French and Spanish that I knew I couldn't do worse in Chinese. As a matter of fact, I received an A.

My instructor said, "Elizabeth, you think like the Chinese."

I had attended a weekend seminar on self-hypnosis before classes began. During the relaxation training session, the instructor had told us to visualize something we wanted. I thought it would be marvelous if I could receive A's in my Chinese and physics classes. I was told to relax, and then to visualize two A's on a blank board.

I'll never know whether the self-hypnosis was the reason for my good grades. But I do suspect that it erased fear I might have felt in my classes and while taking examinations. I enjoyed my courses immensely, and they opened new doors of knowledge for me that will never be closed.

One summer after we moved to Washington, I took my first long vacation along—two weeks in Bermuda. I wrote a poem while I was there.

> The world does not move by force
> but by attraction, not by propulsion
> but by yearning. The world moves by
> love.

# CHAPTER 9

## INTRODUCTION TO THE CHILDREN

To keep step with the song of childhood and not let its shadow mislead you, to let freedom of the human spirit become a passion and truth its foundation stone—these are things I felt strongly about while raising my children.

Now that the children are grown it is hard for me to tell whether I brought them up—or they me. I am prejudiced where my children are concerned. Their strength, tenacity, ingenuity, courage, kindness, and thoughtfulness all speak for themselves.

I will let the following chapters tell their stories. The chapters on and by the children are each different, both in content and format, because each child is different. The children wrote, recorded, or advised on their own chapters.

All of the children were born in good health; they had regular yearly medical checkups with pediatricians and dentists. They were physically well coordinated. They all started the first grade by the age of six and continued on to higher education. Two received master's degrees in the communications fields of speech pathology and information retrieval. One received a bachelor's degree in art. One is a carpenter and writer. The youngest has just received a bachelor's degree in biology.

I thought for years that I had the perfect dyslexic lab. Four out of five of my children couldn't read until they were much older than the average student because they are hereditary dyslexics. My third child, Ellie, was a reader, and for twenty years she was my control; but when Ellie was in her late twenties, we found out that she too was a mild dyslexic. She reads beautifully and enjoys the rhythm of written words and the "decoding" of them, but she had some difficulty in remembering what she had read and in being able to pull out the main theme.

Richard, the youngest, has the most words in his chapter because he had the most difficulty in learning to read.

Perhaps a picture is worth a thousand words.

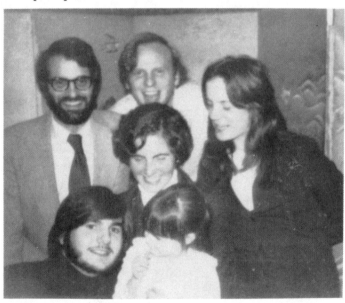

Tom, George, Ellie
Liz
Richard, Tom's daughter Nora

CHAPTER 10


ELIZABETH ("Liz")


Liz, my eldest child, was born in Boston, Massachusetts. She started public kindergarten when we moved to Sewickley, Pennsylvania. Liz liked school, but by the third grade we received reports that her reading was not up to grade average and she would have to repeat the third grade. She has written what she remembers of this early period.


**Mom, she knew best. The outside world understands the physically handicapped, the blind, the deaf, the crippled, the mentally retarded, but not the invisibly handicapped dyslexic.**

**The first child is the perfect one, born with curls on her forehead and two front teeth. People walking along the street used to stop and say, "What a beautiful child."**

**Time for me to enter kindergarten. Mom got scared. I could feel it. Maybe all she could remember was her troubled times through school. My first day of school she spent in the nurse's office, crying. Mom had to relinquish responsibility for education to someone else. This hurt her deeply. Perhaps her whole life just kept flashing in front of her. The**

frustrations and anguish of formal education. All those words to learn to spell, in that funny way, according to Webster. "God, please be with her. Thank you."

When I was six, the family gathered for a summer vacation in Jamestown, Rhode Island. To me, summer vacation meant following the adults. My mother was the first to be married and I was the first grandchild. I was a spectacle to be admired and praised, but not to be listened to or allowed to get in the way of my aunts, grandmother, and mother.

How was I supposed to entertain myself out of earshot of "adult talk?" I trotted off to the kitchen. Grandmother had cookbooks with pretty pictures. One by one, I skimmed through them. Only fifteen minutes had passed. By my grandmother's tone of voice, I knew my disappearing act had to last for at least an hour.

*The Fannie Farmer Cookbook* had a nice picture of tea and cake being served on a silver tray. I knew how to make tea. The recipe for the cake looked easy. I could read and understand the ingredients. I was so smart that I didn't need to read the recipe's instructions. Quietly, I walked into the living room, remembering my manners.

"Excuse me, Mother. May I bake a cake?"

The conversation must have been very interesting, because Mother said, "O.K." No further questions or comments were forthcoming.

I placed the bowls and ingredients on the table. Measuring cup, teaspoon, and tablespoon I translated into coffee cup, little spoon, and big spoon.

I pulled over the chair that children were allowed to stand on to watch or to play in the sink. I took the coffee cup and dug into the flour. One large cup of flour was carefully lifted into the bowl. A small voice kept saying, "Grandmother doesn't like messy kitchens." Two small spoons of baking powder were added. "One-fourth cup of butter." "What does that mean?" I wondered. I decided to leave that problem till last. Into the mixing bowl went a coffee cup of sugar, half a coffee cup of milk, half a small spoon of vanilla, and one egg.

Carefully, remembering the small voice, I stirred with a large spoon. The butter problem returned. I shoved it aside and a new problem appeared—cake pan.

"Excuse me, Mother. What does, one-fourth cup of butter, mean? Also, what pan can I put into the oven?" The adult conversation stopped cold.

"What are you doing, dear?" my grandmother inquired.

"Baking a cake."

"But who said you could?"

"Mother."

"Use any pan that can go on top of the stove for a cake pan, and use the popcorn oil for butter," was my mother's answer.

The problems were solved. I happily went back into the kitchen, added popcorn oil to the mixture, and found a large pan.

Into the oven went my cake. I put the water on the stove for tea. Now where did I find a silver tray? I found an old aluminum tray, washed it, and covered it with aluminum foil. It looked just as pretty and shiny as the picture. Cups and saucers, tea bags, sugar and cream, spoons, and napkins I arranged on the shiny tray, trying my best to have it look like the picture. The cake smelled done. I found the broom and, as I had seen my mother do, took a piece of straw from it, opened the oven door, pulled the pan out with the dishtowel, and stuck the straw into the center of the cake. It came out clean.

The tea water was boiling, and the cake was done. Time for the adult tea party and lots of praise.

I arranged the tea and cake on the foil-covered tray and tried to lift it. The picture did not let me know how heavy water and cake can be for a six year old. My mother came to the rescue. My job was to announce to the adults, "Teatime." My mother carried the tray behind me and placed it on the coffee table. Grandmother asked me to serve the tea. I asked my mother to serve the cake. My aunts were delighted at the pie-shaped cake without icing. My grandmother tasted the cake and warned the others that it was delicious.

The cake was not too sweet, and the adults ate the whole thing. The tea was drunk. The praise was forthcoming. My grandmother considered me smart for being able to read the cookbook. Little did she know that I was reading only one word at a time. The ingredients are nouns. Nouns are the first words a child can learn to read and understand. Mother never considered that I was unable to read the instructions in the recipe.

My aunts were delighted at the excuse to break their diets. My mother was delighted to have the praise of her mother and sisters for her little girl. I was delighted to be included in adult time.

In the third grade, the horror began, just as Mom had feared. "Your daughter's reading is not up to third grade level. Although her math is within normal limits, her spelling and writing ability are definitely not at the third grade level," reported the teacher. "I am not promoting Liz to the fourth grade."

Mom must have thought, "Fear of failure, fear of repeated frustration at the printed word. Now, fear of humiliation at repeating the third grade, in the same public school, with the same teacher. All her friends are being promoted. They will make fun of Liz. How can I hide her from the outside world just a little longer? I know, if it is possible, she will find the strength to live with her reading disability. She will be able to educate others so that she will not be laughed at."

I changed schools. Off to a private school, Sewickley Academy, for the third grade. I enjoyed the dogs the teachers were allowed to bring to class, the lunches and the snacks. Best of all I was enrolled in shop. My worst subjects were still English and spelling. An elderly gentleman tutored me at school.

One day Mom asked me, "What have you learned?"

I answered, "I bring the English grammar book to the room. The tutor sits at the end of a long table. I sit at the other end and read the book. If the word is mispronounced, I am to spell it and he says the word. Never am I asked a question about the passage or if I understand the mispronounced word. I just stumble over words for thirty minutes.''

Anger and frustration grew. The relinquishing of responsibility for education was not working. The educators were not completing their pact. Mom decided that she would have to be the educator and that the educators would be the backup.

Out came the cookbooks and directions for cleaning, laundry, and anything else that Mom could think of to have me read. She would put her finger under each word and move it along as I read. The words I didn't know she would pronounce and explain to me. I cooked and made bread with Mom's help.

Time was set aside after school for us to talk about anything and everything we could imagine or think about. We laughed a lot. We talked about the silly things that happened in school—the teachers who were more interested in how smoothly I read than in how well I understood what I read. I would talk about things I had noticed or was thinking about while we made bread and read cookbooks. Mother would listen and share with me the concepts she was learning in her books.

Little Liz transferred to public school in the seventh grade, after the divorce.

Liz has always had the ability to be self-motivated and inner-directed. An early example of this occurred that summer. In previous summers the family had belonged to a private swimming club. One morning, Liz came down the stairs in her bathing suit, hat, and sunglasses, carrying a beach bag.

She announced, ''I'm going to the club.'' She was only twelve, and I thought she didn't realize that we were no longer members of the swimming club.

But when I said, ''We don't belong to a club any more,'' Liz answered back, ''Oh yes I do!''

With that she went to the backyard and placed a chair next to the baby pool. She sat down, took a magazine out of her beach bag, and proceeded to read.

The rest of us soon followed suit; putting on our bathing suits and sunglasses, we followed Liz to the backyard. From then on our backyard was known as the Club.

Liz would come home from school with full accounts of her fellow students, from the clothes they wore to the way they talked. She moved right along with her studies. Mathematics was her best subject, until she took European history. During the section on the French Revolution she did so well that the teacher asked her to lecture to the class.

I asked her one day, "Why do you have this feeling for the French Revolution?" She answered, "Because I feel like I was there." I asked if she felt like Marie Antoinette. She said, "No, like Madame Defarge. I can just see myself going to the executions and knitting."

In high school, Liz began the aptitude tests for college. At the same time, she was making observations on her own. She did not want to be a check-out girl at the grocery store because she might transpose the numbers. She couldn't be a secretary because her spelling was poor. She said that her only answer was to go on to college. Her SAT scores were not that high, but with the aid of her counselor, she chose a small midwestern women's college, Lindenwood, St. Charles, Missouri.

Liz's work references were remarkable. She had saved up one thousand dollars, earned by baby-sitting over the years. She had five hundred volunteer hours at a hospital and three years as a den mother to a cub scout troop at a home for crippled children. She was also head of the youth group at our church. She was an excellent speaker and organizer.

When asked by her counselor what she wanted to take in college, she answered psychology. The counselor pointed out that one would need a doctorate in the field in order to work as a professional.

At college, to her delight, she found the field of speech pathology. She was fascinated to learn how the tongue works in the mouth. Here was a profession concerned with communication—one person with another. No printed word was needed to communicate; the spoken word was what was important. Liz graduated from Lindenwood with a major in speech and psychology and a minor in mathematics. After two years in the Peace Corps, in Africa, she returned to college and received her master's degree in speech pathology from Catholic University, Washington, D.C.

Elizabeth is now a speech pathology consultant for the Frost Center, Rockville, Maryland, and has started her own catering service, *Mangeon Nous*.

# CHAPTER 11

## THOMAS

Thomas, my oldest son, was born in Philadelphia. He is the Director of the Department of Commerce Law Library. He has been an advisor to the White House library under two administrations. He received a master's degree in Library Science in 1972. Thomas has written the following:

**This is a brief description of my long and difficult struggle in learning how to read. It must be remembered that the difficulty in reading was a definite hindrance to my total learning process because most of the information that a student is expected to learn is acquired by reading. Historical details may not necessarily be correct. Rather, these are my impressions of events and their effect on my reading development.**

**I do not remember when it was that I discovered that I was dyslexic. From the first grade I knew that I had some learning problem and that it derived from my inability to read or comprehend the printed word.**

For me printed symbols were not stationary, but three-dimensional and freely floating on the page. Letters appeared as three-dimensional entities and would revolve independently. Therefore, I could not discern a *b* or *d* from a *p*. I could not fathom how to tell the difference between these three letters. In addition, the order of the letters was not stationary. To this day I can type *eht* and not recognize that it should be *the*.

The result was that I had an extremely difficult time learning to read. However, I realized that I did not have any difficulty in understanding or recalling any other visual or auditory information. In order to compensate for my reading difficulties, I relied on and greatly increased my information gathering through seeing and hearing.

From the first through the third grade my reading became more and more difficult. From almost the first day of the first grade I fell behind most of my classmates in reading because I had great difficulty in comprehending how to translate the printed words into sounds. The letters were not stationary in my mind. They floated, making reading impossible. Slowly I learned to make the letters stationary in my mind, but by that time I had fallen so far behind in my reading skills that I was not able to catch up.

A major secondary problem was that all my teachers realized that I had problems reading and therefore they never called on me to read in class. I feel strongly that, if the teachers had called on me to read more in class, I would have learned to read more quickly.

My third grade teacher left many unpleasant memories with me. She had a way to punish "dummies." She made them sit in the back of the class and never called upon them. This only added to a major problem I have; I am nearsighted. For as long as I can remember, I have only been able to see what is written on a blackboard if I am sitting in the front of the room. It was amazing to be able to see things in the distance.

I confused the teacher by being one of the best students in the class in math. This forced her to switch me from the back of the room to the front when we had math. This was invaluable to my continuing to excel in math, because I could read the blackboard from the front of the class.

I did not successfully complete my third grade and was required to repeat it. [My third grade teacher said that I would be lucky if I graduated from the sixth grade.] The second year in third grade was extremely easy for me because we had material almost identical to that which we had had in the first year. In addition, I had a different teacher, who really tried to help me. I continually amazed her by remembering information that I had collected auditorially from my earlier classes.

My first successful breakthrough came about by accident. I had access to a large collection of smut magazines that had all the pictures torn out of them. I correctly reasoned that the printed words would give me the same tantalizing impressions as the pictures. This brought on my first real desire to read.

During the same summer I went to Laughlin Clinic, in Sewickley, which had just opened to help students with reading problems. The teachers were excellent and they enabled me to accumulate the basic skills that I needed to read. As a consequence I learned how to read in one summer. I also discovered why people read and write: to communicate with another person by means of the printed word. This is not that profound, but for me it explained why it was important to be able to read. I also discovered that, with the proper use of words, this communication can be beautiful and compelling.

I finally had the desire to read and the fundamentals required to read, but there were two problems that carried over from not having been able to read for such a long time. Firstly, I was far behind my classmates in information received from reading. Later, by reading a great deal, I was able to overcome this problem. Secondly, I had great difficulty in spelling. I could not understand why I had to spell words that I could not read. Also, the problems with my three-dimensional perception of the letters and the words made it extremely difficult for me to tell if I had spelled the word correctly. The only way I have learned to spell is by unrelenting practice.

Not until the summer of 1963, when I was fifteen, could I read with any speed. A friend of the family asked me to be a traveling companion on a tour of Canada and Alaska. Two other members of the tour, retired English teachers, helped me a great deal with increasing my reading speed and comprehension. The basic principle was to read something that you wanted to, and slowly increase your speed without going back over what you had read. After you had read a passage, summarize it. This simple method worked extremely well for me. As a result I was able to read and comprehend at a greater and greater speed.

In junior high school we had study hall. I really hated it. One of the few ways to get out of study hall was to work in the library. This was the beginning of a lifetime love affair with libraries and information management, which led to my profession as a law librarian. In addition, I discovered that libraries were a large mechanism for collecting, arranging, and disseminating information. The more I worked in libraries, the more I found out that information is power, and that it can be used to help people. My work with libraries really enforced the fact that it was imperative to be able to read and write.

My tenth grade teacher encouraged me to read more complicated books. My first hard assignment was to read *Dr. Zhivago*, by Boris Pasternak. My teacher made me rewrite the book report four times and in the process showed me how to interpret and appreciate the various levels of meaning of a book. This appreciation of writing led me to a great love of books and the beauty of the printed word.

In the summer of 1966 my grandmother took me on a trip to Europe. During this trip she was horrified at the boring books that I was assigned to read for school. She showed me how to read for sheer enjoyment. "Never waste your time reading a boring book," she used to say.

By the time I reached college I was reading very well, but my problem with spelling and writing was holding me back. Fortunately, I had a wonderful friend, Cindy, who would proofread my papers. She would also show me what I was doing wrong. However, in the first semester of my senior year I came to the conclusion that I was just spinning my wheels and not really getting an education. My advisor said that I was doing fine, but that I should spend more time improving my spelling and writing. He said that I was having problems with these things, but that by no means was I the only one. In fact, there were many students who were in worse shape than I. He said that it was excellent that I was aware of my problem because this is the first step in trying to correct it.

My grandfather suggested that I write a letter a day for practice. I found this to be an excellent way to practice my writing. Unfortunately, I have not kept the habit of writing a letter a day, but I usually now have to write a report every day. In modern education the idea of unrelenting practice of writing is not viewed favorably, but I have found that this is the only way to learn how to communicate effectively in writing.

Twice since then I have thought that my writing was going to "do me in." The first time was in graduate school. I had to take Introduction to Law and Equity, which included the legal writing class. The professor stated that after reviewing the first writing assignment he usually had to require some of the law students to take a fundamental writing class. I was afraid that I would be required to take this class and that it would kill my chances of graduating in one year.

As it turned out, I was not required to take the class. I went to the professor and asked him why. He laughed and showed me some of the papers that were not acceptable. I was amazed at the poor quality of the writing and the spelling, and I realized that I could and did write better than those students.

The second time was after working for eight years. I was required to take a writing class that was being offered by the Department of Commerce. Every management person was required to attend. I was afraid again. As it turned out, the only criticism the instructor gave me was that, in writing a report, both the introduction and the conclusion should be put in the first paragraph instead of the conclusion being put at the end of the report. During the individual discussion period alone with the instructor after the class, most of my time was spent explaining how I had learned to read and write, being dyslexic.

The only time my spelling could have led to problems is in my use of computers. With a computer you have to spell the words correctly or the computer will be searching for the wrong word. This can be an extremely expensive mistake. But I have found that, being aware of my problem in spelling, I have been very careful, and if I do not know how to spell a word, I find out. As a result I have found that, compared with other users, I am extremely effective in the use of computers.

I would like to pass on a few suggestions concerning reading and writing. These are from a dyslexic point of view and are intended for the dyslexic, but they would apply to any person who is trying to learn how to read and write.

The best way to help me to learn how to read was to make me want to read. I am not suggesting that everyone should start with smut magazines, but rather that the books should be interesting, and not the dull, dry, Dick-and-Jane type books.

I have found that my own children are able to read before the first grade and that their books are far more interesting than Dick and Jane. They have a good story and also expose the child to new concepts. A good example of this type of book is *Charlotte's Web*, by E. B. White, which is extremely entertaining and also exposes the child to the concept of death and how to deal with it.

Once you have learned how to read, it is easier to write and spell. You see how the authors write and how the words are spelled. Then practice and more practice in your own writing and spelling will enable you to improve your abilities in effective communication. Perhaps you can find some person who will be good enough to go over your writing and spelling. I have learned most about spelling and writing while on my job because I have to communicate almost daily by writing.

I asked Tom what was one of his most painful memories of school. He said that he remembered one—but would rather have forgotten it. I mention it in detail here because it illustrates how the parent can be a positive and reassuring influence for the child. Thomas was in the third grade, and Valentine's Day was coming soon. He had saved his money and bought all his classmates valentine cards. He addressed each card and took them to school on Valentine's Day. When I saw him after school I asked him how his friends had enjoyed their cards. He told me that his teacher had seen the envelopes and taken them from him. She had copied all the names off the envelopes onto the blackboard. When the class was assembled she had asked all the children to look at the blackboard and see how funnily Tom had spelled their names.

I told Tom that the teacher's actions were inappropriate and that she had also been very rude. I reassured him that he had done the right thing in taking the valentines to school for his friends and that the teacher had been wrong, in this case, to make fun of his spelling. Not only had she shown inappropriate behavior, but also the whole point of the gift of a valentine had been missed.

Thomas said, "Over the years as a child, the thing I felt most strongly about was alienation. The problem of hereditary dyslexia will in time take care of itself. It's the feeling of being alienated from one's peer group and being denied the chance to learn that is the dreadful stigma, a stigma that the student might never outgrow."

One summer Thomas had a job at the National Cathedral, in Washington, D.C. The head of the library asked Tom if he repaired books.

"Of course I do," he answered, not knowing that John Chalmers was referring to rare books rather than to just old books.

Thomas devised a technique for repairing books. He used glue, but he injected it with a hypodermic syringe rather than using the old method of slicing the corners of the binding with a razor blade and inserting the glue with a pointed object.

Thomas also found out how to spell a difficult word in the middle of the night when a paper was due the next day. He found that he could call the long-distance operators if he was stumped (in those days they were not too busy at night) and ask them to help him spell the word. They were delighted to have someone to talk to and gave him the correct spelling. He also found out that the mailman was a good speller. Most people don't realize that one of the troubles in looking a word up in the dictionary is that you have to know how to spell the first part of the word correctly or you are out of luck. For example, *neutral* sounds like "nutral" and *sure* sounds like "shur."

Thomas graduated from the Maret School, in Washington, D.C., and then attended Rockford College, in Illinois. Upon graduation he entered Case Western Reserve University, in Cleveland, Ohio. He received his master's in library and information science in twelve months.

## CHAPTER 12

## ELLANOR ("Ellie")

My second daughter, Ellie, was born in Lancaster, Pennsylvania. She is a mild hereditary dyslexic, but was not diagnosed as such until she was twenty-nine. She was my reader. As a baby she looked different from her siblings. She was bald, round, and cuddly and started nursing on the day of her birth.

When Ellie was a year-and-a-half old, she fell off a second floor porch and narrowly missed hitting the sidewalk below; she landed in the wet mud instead. We rushed her to the hospital, where she stayed for two weeks under observation. She had sustained a hairline crack in her skull. She also had the largest black eye the hospital staff had ever seen. She was pumped full of vitamins, and all ended well.

When she came home she was no longer a quiet, shy child, but let her wishes and thoughts be known. She became an extrovert. She is right-eye dominant now; perhaps the two weeks with her injured left eye shut tightly brought this about. Ellie has never had any trouble with reading.

How Ellie learned to read I do not know. The following are certain things that she did that the other children did not.

She went to a play-school for three years. It was run by a particularly gifted and loving woman. The children played on climbing bar a good deal but spent nearly an hour and a half each day painting with brushes and easels. The easels were in an upright position, so that the child painted at eye level while standing. I remember the teacher saying, "Ellie paints more pictures and goes to the bathroom more than any child I have ever had."

Ellie went to public school. She came home from the first grade one day very excited.

"I learned how to read today," she said. She went to the long kitchen windows and wrote her new words in the condensed moisture on the cold windowpanes—*boy* and *girl*. She did that for the rest of the winter. It was so cold outside that the heat and steam from the kitchen kept the panes foggy with moisture.

I have a theory about this. I feel that Ellie stumbled upon a system of self-teaching, a way to reinforce her new learning of words—*not* by copying long lists of words holding a pencil, but by directly stimulating some part of her brain. *Reproducing the new words by planting and then moving her index finger on a cold sheet of glass*. This tactile approach to word learning provides the student with active physical participation in the use of word forms.

On the other hand, the use of an instrument (pencil or pen) to produce a word requires all kinds of physical messages to and pressure recognitions by the brain. For example, "Hold on to the pencil!" "Don't let it drop!" "You are pressing too hard!" "You're not pressing hard enough!" You are being taught how to use a pencil, not how to recognize a written word!

A friend asked, "Why not use a hot sheet of glass instead of a cold one?" I shuddered at the suggestion! Dyslexics need to be understimulated—cooled down if you like. They are usually taking in too much extraneous information, contrary to what is often thought.

I feel that dyslexics, using both sides of the brain at the same time to gather and tabulate information, have no way to tune out extraneous stimuli. This can be an asset for the dyslexic. They may perceive things that nondyslexics miss. But it makes it very difficult when he or she is young—and trying how to learn to read and write.

One Christmas, Ellie received a rhyming book by Doctor Seuss. Ellie loved to read anything that rhymed. She had a tremendous sense of rhythm and excellent physical coordination. Whether they had played rhyming games and danced at her earlier play-school, I don't know. It has been said that poems give energy; perhaps this is so.

Ellie was a good enough reader to help Thomas with his homework and reading assignments. The only bad mark she received on her report card was for her habit of humming quietly to herself while working in class. They said this disturbed the other children—but perhaps it helped Ellie in some unknown way.

In the third grade I asked that she be held back a year. She was a C student and I was afraid that she might have trouble, as her brother and sister had had, and that to have to repeat a grade later on would be traumatic for her. When I discussed my fears with her school principal, he reassured me, "Ellie is doing just fine. She is physically strong. She belongs with her peer group and she is able to kep up scholastically with her classmates."

Ellie had the same classmates throughout grade school. When it was time for her to go to junior high school she was very excited. However, on the first day she came home in tears, crying as though her heart were broken.

"What's the matter, Ellie?" I asked.

"I'm not with my friends any more. The school has put me in the slow section—with all the bad kids. What have I done wrong? Everybody is making fun of me!"

I made an appointment to see the junior high school principal that afternoon at the school.

"Why was Ellie put in another class, away from all her old friends? She feels as if she is being punished or has done something wrong," I said. "Why has the school done this?"

The new principal was rather young. He stood very straight, perhaps to make himself look more important while he spoke to me.

"Ellie is being put into the slower section to teach her a lesson. She has good potential and has not used it. She is only doing C work in school, and we feel this will jar some sense into her—make her work harder. She can get better grades than C's. When she does, we will put her back with her old classmates. We feel that this change will motivate her to do better work."

I explained the principal's attitude to Ellie. She listened but I don't think she was convinced. When her report card came for the first quarter, there were her usual C's. Ellie didn't work any harder at school and she had less intellectual challenge. She spent a lot of time and energy changing her behavior so she would fit in and be accepted by her new classmates. She stayed an average C student, in that lower section, throughout junior high school. Obviously, high grades had never been as important to Ellie as acceptance by her peers.

To occupy her mind, Ellie began to do a lot of extra reading on her own—science fiction books that she heard about from *The New York Times* book reviews, and anything else she could get her hands on. Once she tried to give a book review on a new book, *The Invisible Man*, by Ralph Ellison, a black author. Her teacher gave her an F and said that there was only one book with the title *The Invisible Man*, and that was written by H. G. Wells. He wouldn't even allow her to bring her book to school to prove her point. She was now being stereotyped as a slow student only because she had been placed in the slower section. Was no one in that section supposed to be able to read a *New York Times* book review?

After graduating from high school, Ellie went to college. She has this to say about her college years.

"I continued in college with average grades. After my sophomore year I left for two years. Not until I decided for myself that I would return to college and work for my bachelor's degree did I make straight A's. I had finally found the field that I was interested in, art. Art was like play for me. It felt like being back in kindergarten.''

Ellie received her Bachelor of Fine Arts degree in studio arts from Jacksonville University. After working for a newspaper for two years, she returned to college for a year to take architectural drafting. She is now living happily in Nantucket, Massachusetts, and working as a layout artist for the newspaper, *The Inquirer and Mirror*.

## CHAPTER 13

## GEORGE

George, my fourth child and second son, was born in Pittsburgh, Pennsylvania. He had excellent health, tremendous energy, and a sense of curiosity.

I read stories to him when he was little, hoping that he would not have the same problem with reading that two of my older children had had.

George started the third grade when we moved to Bethesda, Maryland. He came home from school one day very excited.

"I've learned how to read with my fingers."

He picked up a book and, putting his fingers under the words, began to read aloud. It was the first time that he had ever volunteered with enthusiasm to read to me. I was delighted.

The next day I asked him how his reading was coming along.

His face fell and he said, "My teacher says that only babies use their fingers when they read."

George's reading fell more and more behind. His younger brother, Richard, was also having trouble at school. I took both boys to an eye doctor. The doctor said that the boys' eyes were all right but suggested that I take Richard to a child psychiatrist.

After testing Richard first, the child psychiatrist called George in. Then it was my turn to go into the doctor's office.

He gave his diagnosis. "Richard, George, and you are dyslexic. It is a hereditary trait in your family."

At last, after all those years, I had an explanation why Elizabeth, Thomas, my brother, and I had had so much trouble learning to read.

Trying to find more information on dyslexia, I went to the medical library of the National Institutes of Health. Dyslexia wasn't catalogued at the time. I did find some books, and one of these led me to the Orton Dyslexia Society. This was the only professional group that was of any help to me during this period; the members were most supportive. It was fun to go to the large meetings. It was nice to know that I was not alone.

Fortunately, by the time George was ready for the fifth grade there were enough boys his age with similar reading problems to form a special class. It was called Catch-up Class.

George said, "The boys are very competitive but it is a good experience."

During the summer George played football. Both he and Richard signed up for Y.M.C.A. day camp. It provided swimming, art, and crafts. Each received a good report at the end of the summer.

George was becoming a leader. He knew everyone and questioned everyone, teachers and students alike. He had received the nickname Flamingo. He had light red hair, blue eyes, and like his sister Ellie, excellent coordination.

In the sixth grade, during the Vietnam War, George came home from school one day and told me how he would direct the U.S. Navy ships in the Pacific if he were in command—and explained his reasons. I later asked his godfather, Jack Lauritzen, what the ability to take on such an all-encompassing concept was. He told me it was logistics (the procurement, distribution, maintenance, and replacement of materiel and personnel).

One summer there were riots in Washington, D.C., and people feared they would spread out to the suburbs. The women in the neighborhood talked about what we should do. It was decided that, if there were trouble, George would be put in charge of the little children and would take them down to the woods, where there were tunnels. We knew George was familiar with the tunnels and would be able to lead the children to safety.

By the seventh grade George was back in the mainstream class at the junior high school. He spent the next two years there.

By the end of the eighth grade it was evident he was in serious need of help with his reading. The decision was made to send him as a boarder to the Kildonan School for boys, in New Jersey. It was run by Diana King, who was considered to be one of the top people in the field of teaching dyslexic children to read. George said Mrs. King told him after a year and three months, "George, I have taught you all I can. All you have to do is to start using it." He came home and was enrolled in high school.

When he graduated, physics was his best subject. Speech class was a natural for him, but he did not prepare his lectures well. However, he had no trouble ad-libbing for twenty minutes in front of the class. His reading was still slow, so he relied heavily on his memory. He also enjoyed history.

While he was in Nantucket visiting his father, friends encouraged him to go on to college, even though his SAT score and grade point average were low. That fall he enrolled at Towson College as a night student to try to get a high enough grade point average to qualify as a day student.

During this period, I was attending Montgomery College. One day, during a ride home from an off-campus lecture, one of my classmates commented, "You live near George Fleming."

"Yes," I responded, "he is my son."

"Oh, that explains a lot!" my classmate said, and we both laughed.

One of the other students in the car asked, "Who is George?"

My classmate replied, "He was a classmate of mine in high school who had an I.Q. of 135 and didn't know it."

At age twenty, George went to Europe for a six-week summer course organized by the Richmond School of Economics. He had the opportunity to speak with leading economists and advisors for the European Common Market. He also attended lectures at the London School of Economics. He was introduced to the world of international banking. The trip covered nine countries.

The next year he began to study commercial real estate in Washington, D.C., taking courses at the American University and at Maryland night school.

After a year and a half, his grandfather made him an offer, "If you'll go to college full time, I will take on your expenses." George accepted. It took a lot of courage because he had to start from the beginning as a daytime freshman.

He has said that friends have taught him everything he has learned in school, even how to read, and that his grandfather taught him mathematics. He has taken courses in philosophy and accounting, as well as the required freshman and sophomore courses. He is working toward a degree in systems analysis.

George once spoke of a method I used to help him: "When I would come home from school so frustrated because of my school environment and my inability to control it, you used to listen to me, then help me stimulate my mind with some other subject or some other point of view so that I could rise above it. You used to give me big lectures, too, on *personal integrity*—on fighting for what I thought was right. You told me to stand behind what I said or did because, if I did not, I would lose a part of myself, and none of us are so big that we can afford to do that."

This year George took a leave of absence from the big city and the large academic environment and is living in Nantucket, Massachusetts, where he is working as a carpenter and writing.

George wrote the following poem which was published in the *Inquirer and Mirror*.

## The Clarification

The clarification...my love
is the sharing of one heart
to one heart, one soul to one
soul.

The soft touch of your hands
around your heart shows me the
wonderful person you are
and it brings joy into my
life.

My soul is of my substance
and it is the treating of each
other as though we were gods
to one another.

My words are of truth, time
and thought.

Love to me is the sharing of
one heart to one heart, and
one soul to one soul.
The dream of my life I share
for one night.

Phantom of my life

George says this of dyslexics: "A dyslexic thinks in a circle or wheel—going from the perimeter toward the center or goal. This does not imply thinking in circles but rather approaching a subject from many different points of view simultaneously. The average person thinks in a straight line. The dyslexic circles the subject and ends in the center."

## CHAPTER 14

## RICHARD

John Richard, my youngest child and third son, was born in Pittsburgh, Pennsylvania. When he was twelve months old, I called the other children into the kitchen and told them that I wanted to have a conference. We sat around the kitchen counter, and I told them about a lecture I had heard the night before, "The Seven Steps of Emotional Development of the Child."

"The child must have a sense of trust before he is eighteen months old," I said. "We have only six more months to be able to help Richard develop trust. Do you think you can help him?"

They all answered yes.

That was the first of many family conferences to come. The children entered into the spirit of the assignment. A precedent was set that day. In the future, any of us could call a family conference. I needn't have worried. Richard had no trouble with trust. He knew that we loved him and were taking good care of him.

Richard had three bronchial attacks before he was a year-and-a-half old. I had read an article in *Reader's Digest* about a mother who had spoken to her son while he was in a coma for three weeks at a hospital. When the child came out of the coma, he told his mother he had heard her voice as she spoke to him and he remembered what she had said to him. I decided to try this with Richard's bronchial problem.

I went into Richard's room one night while he was asleep. I picked him up gently so as not to wake him and started speaking to him. I asked him to please forgive me for "fouling up" so—for the loss of his father, for my being in the hospital while he was a little baby, and for my not being there to love him more. I started to cry, and Richard threw up. There was a tremendous feeling of relief. Richard never had another attack of bronchitis.

By the time he was four he had developed quite a sense of adventure. One day he was gone from the yard and I called the police to report him missing. They asked if he had on any unusual clothing. I answered no. Within the hour the police car drove up, and there was Richard sitting in the back seat with a Mickey Mouse hat on, big ears and all!

Richard entered kindergarten when we moved to Bethesda, Maryland. He was bright and alert. That first Christmas in Bethesda, Santa Claus gave Richard a real piano. His piano playing was remarkable. The piano tuner recommended that we take him to the music department of Catholic University. There they suggested that Richard go on composing his own music, rather than have a piano teacher, because he could not read sheet music. Notes, like the written word, are printed left to right, along straight lines. I was told to go to the library for Richard and check out classical piano records, starting with the early piano composers and working up to the modern ones of today.

Richard would hear Bach and then imitate his style in a new composition of his own. No one else in the family was even interested in classical music. He titled one of his early compositions "The Day after Church" and another "The Day after One." These pieces were filled with emotion and suspense. He developed his own skills, practicing one or two hours every day.

When Richard was in the second grade, he was diagnosed as a hereditary dyslexic. I was advised by the school principal to place him in Special Education because he still could not tell numbers from letters.

His second grade teacher was marvelous. Not so, his third grade teacher. She gave him writing assignments of one sentence, to be written over and over again for two or three days. One sentence was, "My daddy is a good boy." I insisted that she at least give him something worthwhile to copy, pointing out that his father was not a boy, but a man. Once, walking with Richard on his way to school, I asked, "How do you feel about your teacher?"

He said, "She is a nice woman, but she doesn't know how to teach."

I queried, "What would you like to be learning now, Richard?"

He answered, "A poem."

I asked, "Which one?"

He responded, "You know—that one about 'I and be, be, being.' "

"Do you mean that line 'To be or not to be: that is the question.' "

"Yes, that's the one I mean!"

That afternoon, when Richard returned home, I found Shakespeare's *Hamlet* and the soliloquy "To be or not to be." We read it over together and he proceeded to memorize it, line by line. It took him nearly three weeks, but he learned it.

At school, instead of being pleased that he had done so well in his memorization, the school psychologist said that very disturbed people could memorize too. Richard's survival of this type of attitude must have been due to some superhuman strength he possessed—something that came from within himself.

I did not learn until Richard was older that he had always been able to see three aura colors (of the energy field that surrounds the living human body) around people. Perhaps he could read what other people were feeling even if he couldn't read the written word.

When Richard was about ten he came to me and said, "I'm worried, Mother."

"About what?" I asked.

"George and Thomas are so big and I am so little. I'll never be as tall as they are."

George had a full red beard in the eighth grade and Thomas had a rich brown beard he was shaving off every morning.

I felt sorry for Richard, although I certainly wasn't worried about his future growth. To make him feel better I made an appointment with our chiropractor. After checking Richard she said, "Richard is in excellent health. I told him not to worry. He will be taller than either of his brothers." Richard could hardly wait to get home and tell them. They teased him, saying, "We'd better beat you up now while we are still taller than you are!" Indeed Richard did finally grow to be six feet two inches tall.

I always tried to relieve fears and doubts whenever I could. Certainly we all learned in those years that the most important function of a family is to give emotional support and reassurance.

When Richard was in the fourth grade, he was placed back into regular school. Richard and one other child in the county did not fit into any specific classification for learning. A very wise decision was made—to take Richard out of Special Ed, put him back into the mainstream, and give him all the *positive reinforcement* possible. His report card was to be a progress report, with no grades issued.

By junior high school he was taking music appreciation, shop, art, and biology. His biology teacher was a gift from God for Richard. He asked Richard to decide what he would like to study. Richard seized on this opportunity to ask if he could dissect a frog. He was familiar with the idea of dissection because some family friends were doing research for the National Institutes of Health. Some were dissecting worms. The teacher consented and ordered the material. Richard was able to learn by doing.

Richard kept a notebook. I asked to see it. He was keeping notes all right, but the words all ran into each other. I made no comment about his spelling, although it was impossible for me to read his words. But I did suggest that he leave larger spaces between his words, explaining that they would be easier for him to read.

Richard received much help from our public librarian. He had met her often over the years while taking out recordings of classical music. She advised him to apply for a card from the National Library Service for the Blind and Physically Handicapped. He was eligible because of his handicap, dyslexia. Records for the blind, which the Library produces, are called talking books.

During high school, Richard got a summer job working for the National Institutes of Health as a biologist aid. Our family income was low enough to make him eligible for special government employment. It was a most valuable experience.

When he graduated from high school, he was accepted as a boarder at Echard College, Saint Petersburg, Florida.

He did extremely well in music, but he says, "Music will always be my avocation." He lectured on holistic health. He struggled through biology, physics, and chemistry. It sometimes took him longer than ten minutes to read one page of a textbook, but he said, "It's worth it!"

The following has been taken from a tape Richard made of his memories and reflections about school.

**The first difficult time of my life was in school, the second semester of my first year. I realized I was a little bit different from all the rest.**

**There were three or four of us in the slow section. We read different books and worked different math problems. The other children didn't notice the difference, but I did. We talked more than the rest of the class too.**

My second year I went into Special Education with a new teacher. She was fantastic, but the move to Special Education definitely gave me my first feeling of separation because of my difficulties in reading and spelling.

In Special Ed, we had the mentally retarded, physically handicapped, and a lot of troublemakers. This is where I started to be eyed as a real troublemaker.

The teacher did try to expand our reading and writing. But what was most important to our learning was drawing maps. She would say, "Draw your house. Map out the rooms." For us these exercises were fun, and they helped us to understand and record dimensions.

Mrs. Co, our third grade teacher, taught us by set rules and regulations. "You may not read your book using your fingers. You may not chew gum in the class."

At home I was starting to take radios apart. I loved working with electricity. Since I had been a preschooler I had been able to repair plugs and hook up batteries. I kept on trying to learn at home.

I started tutoring with Mrs. Fischer, our Sunday School teacher. I think this upset the third grade Special Ed teacher because she saw a definite improvement. Anytime that I brought up the work I did with Mrs. Fischer, Mrs. Co would knock it down, saying, "Oh you just play around."

Once Mrs. Fischer planned a gift for me to give to my mother as a surprise—my playing the recorder. Playing the recorder was a new experience for me—reading notes. It was new and it was fun! As I was carrying my recorder, Mrs. Co stopped me and said, "Oh, you play the recorder! Let me hear." After I had played my little piece she laughed and said, "It's coming there, but you don't have your beat down yet."

I think back to that time and ask myself, "My God, why, in education, is it so important to point out the *negative* aspects of the student's growth?"

It was nice at this time to have a parent who acknowledged me not just as a child, but as a person. *Home was a place in which I knew I would never be attacked.* It was a place I could go to and not be afraid of problems with writing and spelling, or of being called an "idiot" or "dummy," or of being told, "You can't read! Ha-ha-ha!" Home was a safe place I will always remember.

One night, while I was in Mrs. Co's class, I walked home by myself and I started to cry and cry. I said, "God, if anything, please, *please*, get me out of Mrs. Co's class." Maybe this started my spiritual growth; I was out of the Special Ed program in the fourth grade, the next year.

My fourth grade class was full of all my friends. This was very good for me. There were new learning experiences, especially in the field in which I would end up—science. I found a friend who helped me a lot with spelling and science projects. But then he got sick and was out of school for a month. I'm on my own, I realized. And ever since then I have been on my own.

I got more into music at school. When we sang every Thursday it was one of the biggest things that ever happened in my life. I could *do* something! I could remember the lyrics! I was asked three or four times to lead the group. To me at that age, after all the negative criticism, it was tremendous!

The fourth grade teacher was very helpful, not only in music and the sciences but also in saying, "You are a person. You're *not* a dummy just because you can't read!" She expected me to do just the same amount of work as everybody else did, and if I couldn't do as well, there was no problem.

Someone asked me to read down a list of spelling words.

"I can't do this," I said.

'Sure you can," responded the teacher.

She took me up to her desk with the list of words and we sat down and went through them, splitting them into syllables. After that, I started reading a book, going through and reading by syllables. Then I went back and read the word list to the other students.

This is when I learned to spell the months of the year and the days of the week. Nothing much, but it was my big break. For the first time, instead of someone saying, "You can't do that," someone had said, "*Yes you can* do that."

In the fifth grade everything was independent study, including science. It was just hell.

I had friends then, but they were few and far between. That was the time I was just starting to really notice the opposite sex and that was the big thing for me and most of my other classmates. That was the start of hell-raising times. I started smoking cigarettes [nothing stronger].

In the next year I had a new tutor, Mrs. Hannah, who herself was dyslexic. She knew where my capacities were and pushed them until she couldn't push any more. *It wasn't the negative but the positive push that worked.* Perhaps sometimes I wouldn't have done my homework, or couldn't have done it. All *hell* would break out! I still remember sweating. She would yell at me, "Why didn't you do it?" And this was positive. [I repeat because I think this is important.] She *expected* more of me than most other people had. She expected me to read. She expected me to write. She expected me to learn my grammar.

The next year I had a *choice*: to go on to sixth grade or to transfer to Tilden Junior High School [in an adjacent school district] as a seventh grader. I opted for the seventh grade at Tilden because I wanted to catch up with my own grade.

Tilden was not very well equipped to handle the dyslexic, though it was equipped to handle students with other learning disabilities and it was nearly like a rehabilitation center for emotionally disturbed children. All during my education I think not even the educators knew the differences between the dyslexic student, the emotionally disturbed student, and the student with other learning disabilities.

I was petrified by the new situation, the new school, the new teachers. I wondered, "What will people think of me?"

I told my guidance counselor about my fear. He took me around to see each of my teachers, for me to tell them my story and my fears. He was right to do that. This was a positive experience for me. It was the first time that I was able to communicate with my teachers, my educators, about my concerns and disappointments, and what I wanted to achieve.

English now became fun for me. Before, it had always been very difficult for me. I had not realized that after a certain grade we would study other things besides grammar. We started reading and learning about poets. I was introduced to the plays of Shakespeare, and to public speaking. This gave me good feelings about a subject that had always before been a negative experience.

Also there was physical education. At this time, I was in puberty and I was overweight. In no way did I have a positive image of myself.

I became more dependent on the church. Yet at the same time I realized that this wasn't the only answer. There was something more than just the church. I had more problems than the church could help with.

I tried being helped psychologically at a county clinic. I remember that my mother went with me. Everybody else there was really off his rocker. [Perhaps so was I.] So this clinic was no help whatever. I knew that there was something more.

Finally I started private therapy with Dr. Tom. I refused to tell any of my friends. But, much as I didn't want my friends to know about it, I realized that I very much needed it.

Art was a very positive thing for me. I could really draw trees. The teacher asked me to sit down and draw something, so I drew a tree with a bird. He looked at it and said, "This is unbelievable! This is ninth grade work!"

That was like giving me a shot of speed or whatever pep pills you can think of. It started me off in art. I learned about Van Gogh, Gaugin, and all the others.

In eighth grade I was still overweight by fifteen or twenty pounds. I felt a little funny about it; yet I realized it was all right to feel different. I didn't have to compete! I didn't have to worry about what other people thought of me!

By ninth grade, my old habit of trying so hard to please other people and make friends was gone. I strutted down that hall. I would wistle and kind of tap my feet. People laughed and I laughed back. I didn't feel that I was being made fun of. This was a time I was discovering myself.

In the ninth grade I went to the Special Resources Center, where they were to help me with the reading and whatever else I was interested in. The teacher was very, very good.

The class was for problem students. No one else in the class was a slow reader. This was the heavy bunch—the dope dealers and the gamblers. I was the straight one in the crowd.

The reason this class was so important was that I actually read some of the books. This was amazing for me at that time.

History became fascinating and fun. We would have a lecture or a movie and then discuss it. We had discussions about American Indians and our moral feelings about them. Why did we slaughter the Indians? Which side was really better? We were allowed to bring our emotions and our discoveries into the class.

Then I went to high school. Driver education class was a plus. I was asked to be a driver education assistant! I was able to do something good!

Also, it was important that I was able to tell someone—a teacher—that she was wrong about me. I took a music course and was asked to play one of my pieces on the piano.

The teacher said, "That was fantastic. It's unbelievable how much potential you have! But the beat is all off. The timing is all off."

I said, "I thank you very much for the compliments, but the timing is right." This was the last time I took a class from her!

I started to help out in theater, not at my school but at another high school where my friends from Tilden had gone. I helped build sets and did other jobs. It was fun. It was an activity in which everybody worked and had a good time. No one was competing. It was a group project and it didn't have to do with reading, spelling, or how fast you could run. I guess for those who couldn't hammer a nail straight it was hard, but for me it was yet another positive experience.

In the eleventh grade I worked for the National Institutes of Health as a biologist aid. The important step in this year was working. It was essential to me to be able to support myself. During the summer I also worked, so I got a true feeling for an eight-to-five job.

In my senior year, I knew I was going straight into college when I graduated and I wouldn't be having any real fun time for myself for a while. So I asked if there were any openings for stage crew or lighting and sign crew for the senior spring musical. The teacher in charge suggested, "Why don't you go for tryouts?" He knew my problem with dyslexia and he apparently didn't think much about it. So that's what I did.

This is important because it is a case of learning how to succeed where you feel you can't. You have to believe in yourself. What makes that important is that you then get rid of anxiety.

When I went to the tryouts, I said to myself, "This is going to be fun and I am going to have a good time. Maybe I'm not any good at acting, but anyhow, I want to try. What I really want is to be on the stage crew. I have nothing to lose."

Tryouts were fun. Three people auditioned at the same time. We started dancing, but five steps into the music I stopped because I had forgotten the rest. I turned around and the other two had stopped too.

The guy next to me said, "I can't remember my steps."

I said, snapping my fingers, "It doesn't matter. Just keep the beat."

I started doing my own little kicks. This relieved the pressure. That was important for getting the part because, if I got into the space where I felt it was too important to me that I get the part, I would have the fear of failure.

The following day I was called back. When I went in, I saw the scripts on the stage. My first thought was, "Oh hell. They are going to have us read! What the heck, I'll try anyway!"

So I sat down and started reading the script over and over. I got up on the stage. My first two lines were great—then I got nervous and started dropping my voice and whispering. But I got through it and I did get the part [the senior male lead in *Gypsy*]. Being in the performance gave me satisfaction—and I found that I had stage presence. I mention this because it was a big step—the beginning step—in allowing myself to go away to college.

I couldn't be registered according to my reading level; my vocabulary was so diverse. I couldn't spell some second grade words and yet I could spell some seventh grade words. However, I was accepted to Echard College. This was scary.

Echard had a special program for freshmen. My first semester I started with six courses: chemistry, theater projects, Foundations [an English course], biology, writing skills, and choir. I reassured myself, "You can get through all these courses. Just pass them. You will be doing O.K."

I picked a course called The Magic of Chemistry, thinking possibly we would be learning about chemistry. Fortunately, I was unable to read the class description; this turned out to be the hardest course there was.

The first assignment was to write a page about yourself. I had always written about my dyslexia, so why not this time? When the professor got the paper, he did a double take. He said, "Just try your hardest, Richard."

I did. I worked my hardest for forty hours a week in the library doing research. Doing research, opening up the book and being able to read, *potassium, nitrogen, sodium, phosphorous*, was a big plus for me. And I was doing it on my own. No one at the college contacted me during the term, and the professor was no big help.

My first paper came back from Foundations. It was a three page paper. It got thrown back at me—unacceptable. I looked it over and the spelling was atrocious; but it was readable if you looked at it phonetically.

There was a writing clinic at school. I went there and said, "The only problem I have is with the spelling." The people at the clinic helped me to correct the spelling and then I retyped the paper and submitted it. This time I got a C minus.

In my other courses I was turning in papers once a week. For the theater workshop I was reading [or trying to read] three plays a week and writing about them or a movie we had seen. Writing papers became automatic except for the spelling. The grammar, the organization, and everything else were there. It was the most frustrating time I have ever had.

A point came when I started to slow down. I remember myself saying, "Oh, this is too much!" As soon as I said this, I turned in my first late paper.

I tried to excuse myself but I didn't have to. The instructors just looked at me and said, "Oh you are—what do they call it?—dyslexic or dizzy or something. Don't worry about it. Do it in a week."

But I didn't do the paper in a week. I went back and said, "I don't think I can do it."

"Fine," the instructor said, and that was that.

Later on I thought back, and said to myself, "That's ridiculous! I can do papers. I have been doing fifteen, three to five page, papers up till now." I sat down and composed a paper two-and-a-half pages long on my typewriter. It was nothing dramatic or big, but I did turn it in. I got a B on it.

After this, someone thought up the idea of my taping my papers. This was fine. It helped me with my grammar, my organization, and my oral communications and voice projection skills. But it did not help me with my spelling.

Echard College had admitted seven dyslexics without even knowing what the word *dyslexia* meant. By the end of the semester I was the only one left. The others had dropped out. I was angry and petrified, thinking, "What will happen to me?" But I continued. My first semester I had a 3.1 grade point average!

At the present time in my college career I am working and struggling, and probably will forever, in biology, my major. I have a grade point average of 2.7. This is a drop. But I now take the attitude that it doesn't matter if the grade drops; I'll still go on.

It might take me a little longer than four years to get through college. But I feel it is necessary for me. I am back at the point where I was before the third grade, when I said, "I want to experience. I want to discover." Here at college we have a chance to discover and to experience, not only new subjects and information, but also ourselves.

CHAPTER 15

POSITIVE ADVICE ON PARENTING DYSLEXIC
CHILDREN

> *Sometimes it's better to believe*
> *the heart than all the knowledge*
> > *in the world.*
> > ...unknown

A time came when I had to stop believing the experts and
believe my heart instead. I never considered letting outsiders
tell me my children had damaged I.Q.'s because they couldn't
read. I knew my children. I saw and talked to them. They were
bright, inquisitive, and kind. So what if they couldn't read?

I knew the need to read comes to a hereditary dyslexic
when he or she needs to have more words to express thoughts
or feelings. Four of my children were in their late teens when
this inner need arose. I was thirty-two.

My son George expressed it, "I need to know the words to
communicate my thoughts."

I have found in the parenting of hereditary dyslexic children that it is imperative to be ***optimistic***. Perhaps it would be true in parenting any child. My favorite definition for *optimist* is that the optimist knows how rotten things can be, therefore he is often pleased to see how well things are going. Robert Browning put it, "To dry one's eyes and laugh at a fall, and baffled, get up and begin again."

In raising dyslexic children, as in all of life, what is important is getting up! A child psychiatrist once said, "Getting to the knees before standing, that's what being a Christian is all about." When asked how often he had to do that, he replied, "Sometimes twenty times a day."

I cannot stress enough how important I think it is to surround the dyslexic child with the ***world of ideas***. The dyslexic feeds on ideas the way a normal person feeds on words. The ideas have to become verbalized, and that is the dyslexic's long-term goal.

The brain is like a muscle. Exercise it or it will atrophy. I feel it is preposterous to think that the only way to exercise the brain is to read. There are many other ways—looking, listening, speaking, exploring, and most importantly, thinking.

The purpose of education is to prepare ourselves for the world in which we live. The world of missiles, computers, galaxies, interdenominationalism, splitting of the atom, instant communication, holograms, and lasers is ours. We need to use the information and, more importantly, to understand it.

Not to belittle the three Rs, but there are many other ways to augment learning—for example, movies, television, book records, and conversation. What would have happened to our learning system if the record player had been invented before the printing press?

As a parent I feel a ***sense of humor*** is one of the most important things you can help a child develop. When the children were little I went to the library to find a book on the subject. I could find only one. It was a book on reading which included a comment on children and humor. A child has a sense of humor when it sees something is out of proportion or out of balance—for example, a man with a hat *so big* that, when he puts it on his head, it covers his face. To know when things are out of proportion you must know when things are in proportion. According to the book, a child develops a sense of humor by the age of three-and-a-half or four.

It is most important for the parents of hereditary dyslexic children to keep a sense of proportion. The child will learn to read when he is older—Einstein did, Woodrow Wilson did.

However, the pain of not being able to read is something that most of you will never understand or experience. The emotional and psychic pain of isolation is tremendous. It is bad enough that the child feels this pain. If the parents overreact, it puts a double burden on the child.

To raise hereditary dyslexic children, you must keep track of the larger gestalt (or whole picture)—the long-term goal. Try to keep your own sense of humor. Keep faith. The time does pass. The children do grow up. They do learn how to read. They do become professionals, if they want to.

I feel it is important to help a child develop *a positive self-image* because a child will guard his or her self-image, even if it is a negative one, feeling it is better to have a negative self-image than no self-image at all.

When my children were having trouble reading, I would tell them, "You will learn to read. You just have a problem. English is just like any other language. It takes some people longer than others to learn how to read and write it. For some it is a short-term goal and for others a long-term one. Read cookbooks, road signs, anything. By the time you want to go to college, you will have it under control."

The big question, What do you want to do or be when you grow up? is an important one. I let the children decide for themselves. If their choice was one that would require a doctorate, all right. By thinking about it while they were young, they were able to set up long-term goals. An inner attitude began to develop.

Plenty of people who read well never go to college or find a job. I allowed my children the freedom to dream their own future. It was in the *wanting to* that they found their *inner drive* that made them go on—sometimes against what seemed impossible odds.

Once a hereditary dyslexic has reading under control, anything else is kid's play. Maturation and an inquisitive mind are two of the greatest assets they can have. All my children have shown great tenacity in learning any subject, once interest has been aroused. They seem to motivate themselves.

Another way a parent can help enormously is to expose the children to as many *intellectual activities* as possible, for example, music, theater, and thought-provoking conversations. Help them to enlarge their world and their vocabulary of understood spoken words.

Manners were always very important to me. I was well aware that the children would copy mine. However, one day I couldn't take their early morning fighting any more and called up the stairs, "Cut out that damn fighting! If you must say something to each other in the morning, say 'Good morning,' and that's all." The bickering stopped.

At the breakfast table we would often tell the dreams we had had during the night. The children were a big help to me when I had had a difficult dream. They helped by listening. They would sometimes give their own insights. I only hope that I was as helpful when they told theirs. At least I listened. The dream that came up for nearly all the children was the basic one of wild animals. I suggested that perhaps the animals represented their own "animal drives, " and rather than be afraid of the animals, if they showed up in other dreams, the children should speak to them.

Every morning I would check the television section of the newspaper for good programs—particularly the educational ones. If I found a good program, I would tell the children about it and try to watch it with them. Afterward we would talk about it together.

If I couldn't watch the program, I would ask them to watch it for me, and then ask them questions about it later. "What was the program about? What did you think about it? How do you feel about it?"

We all loved receiving new information. One night we watched a program about the research going on with magnets at Massachusetts Institute of Technology. We were fascinated. It didn't bother any of us that we didn't understand it all. It was fun watching the tremendously large magnetic coils being set up in the laboratory. And it gave the family a shared experience to talk about.

George has asked me to include information on how I handled my children's anger and frustration. When the children were little they sometimes whined, as children will. One day I couldn't stand it. I screamed out at them, "Be angry if you must, but cut out that damned whining! What are you angry about?" Much to my surprise they told me.

It became very important for the children and me to be aware of our own feelings and particularly our anger, when it arose.

The tremendous feeling of frustration at not doing well at school when they were obviously very bright children would sometimes become nearly unbearable. My experience in fighting the school systems all those years wasn't much better. One household remedy we had for rage, anger, or general frustration was to throw bottles against a brick wall outside the house. It was a controlled system in which we could let off steam. No one used it often, but it was a Godsend when we needed it.

When George and Richard were first diagnosed as hereditary dyslexics, I asked the child psychiatrist, "Is there anything I can do to help them with their school work?"

He informed me in no uncertain terms, "It is enough of a job being the mother. Leave the teaching up to the school. Your job is to keep them in good emotional health—and you do that by keeping yourself in good emotional health."

My sister Edythe had once put it to me as a riddle, "How do you have happy children?"

I said, "I don't know."

"Give them a happy mother," she replied. The psychiatrist was now saying nearly the same thing.

Once, I received a telephone call from a Sunday School teacher who threatened to flunk one of my children in Sunday School class because he couldn't read! If you can't read, you can't be confirmed? It was ridiculous! The minister agreed with me. There was no more problem.

One of the most difficult decisions I have ever had to make, I made when George was nine. His Sunday School teacher, Mrs. Fischer, was a reading expert and she said, "I would love to teach George how to read. He is such a bright boy." Richard was still in Special Education and he still couldn't tell his numbers from his letters. George was at least operating in regular school and doing well in math. So I explained to her, "George's brother Richard has a much more severe case of hereditary dyslexia. Can you take both boys?"

She said, "I'm sorry, but I can't."

I asked her, "Please take Richard then, instead of George."

She agreed. Her child was autistic, a teenager. So we made an exchange of time. She would tutor Richard, and I would drive her child to private school each day.

At home I was instructing the children how to use the telephone. My mother had carefully trained me as a child, "Don't hold your mouth too close to the phone! Speak clearly." I taught this to my children. I did such a good job that I ran into trouble one day. A friend, passing me on the street, said, "Why didn't you answer my phone call? Your son took down my name and number." I tried to explain to him that my son couldn't write, so it would have been impossible for him to have written down the message. My friend didn't believe me. He said, "Your son was so businesslike on the phone. He said he was carefully writing my message down and would give it to you."

I dealt with the problem by instructing the younger children, "Ask all callers to telephone me again if I am not at home. Do not take any written messages."

I gave my children reassurance as often as possible. In most cases, this was the only place they were receiving any.

For instance, if I were talking to a friend or on the phone, I would motion them over and hold their hands or touch them in some way so that they would know—I had recognized their wish to speak. Often it was just the touch, the recognition of their presence, that they wanted—a little reassurance that they were noticed.

The point was to let the children know that, although I was busy at that moment, I was not rejecting them. They knew they were next in line and, as soon as there was a break in the conversation, it would be their turn to speak.

I used the same sense of touch when I was trying to talk to the children. If for some reason they were not attentive or were not understanding what I was saying, I could catch and hold their attention if I gently touched them while I spoke to them. Usually we would make eye contact.

Good advice given by my mother was, "Don't ever underestimate a child and don't tell them a lie." My mother had answered nearly every question I put to her in my childhood with, "I'll give you three guesses. What do you think?" I used the same approach with my children when they asked questions like, "What's that?"

Whenever anyone discarded books, the children took turns going through the piles (murder mysteries, reference books, old German bibles, philosophy books). You name it, they took it. Children can love and collect books without always knowing how to read them. It's wanting to read them that counts first.

I've never stinted on paper and I've tried to teach the children not to. Often the habit of writing the words too closely is a cover-up so that no one will notice their poor spelling. If children are able to spell words phonetically, the way they sound, they can usually read them themselves, as long as they leave a large enough space between each word.

Which reminds me that once I asked Jack Lauritzen, the solid-state physicist, "Why do you use so much paper to do a simple calculus problem for me?"

He answered, "It's easier to write down every step; then, if I make a mistake, it is easier to go back and find it."

I was a great believer in creative outlets, for children and adults, and I encouraged all my children to find one. Elizabeth was an excellent cook and enjoyed needlework. Thomas worked with model boats and planes. Ellie sewed. George did leatherwork. Richard did minor electric repairs and played the piano.

Here is a point I feel strongly about. In my experience, all the hereditary dyslexics I have known seem to have extrasensory perception of some sort. I took my ability to feel other people's emotions for granted for years. I thought everyone knew what other people felt. It has recently been pointed out to me that this is not so. This ability is called clairsentience. My children all have it.

I tried to teach the children, "Fight for what you think is right." One example of this was when Tom and two friends asked me if they could set off a *little* toy cannon in our yard on Halloween night. I said yes.

That night Tom didn't come home until after midnight. I was very upset and asked him where he had been. Out came the story. After Tom and his friends had set off the toy cannon, a policeman had come into our yard. He had made them get into the patrol car, and driven them out into the country. He had stopped the car, opened their door, and said to them, "Find your own way home. This will teach you to make loud noises on Halloween!"

I was incredulous. I was furious.

The next morning I told Thomas, "I am going to put in a complaint against the police officer. To take you out of your own yard, without my consent, when I was in the house at the time, is bad enough. But to not formally charge you all at the police station, and instead, at a whim, to take three boys out into the country and leave them, is all wrong."

Then I telephoned the other boys' parents to ask if they were going to do anything about the unwarranted actions of the police officer. Both boys' fathers said they were not going to do anything about it.

I told Thomas, "There are some things in life that you have to fight for, even if it means going to jail."

I telephoned the police captain and made an appointment for him to see Thomas and me. With some fear and trembling, on my part at least, Tom and I walked down to the police station.

As so often happens in these cases, it turned out pleasantly. The police chief was there with his son, the officer who had taken the boys. He had just been helping the police out on Halloween and he was not a real policeman. That was why he had not followed police procedure properly. He apologized to Tom and me.

A few years ago I heard joke lines were being passed around by some postgraduates at California Institute of Technology. "This is one of my more dyslexic days." "I think I'm feeling dyslexic today."

The difference was that for them it was a temporary state. For the hereditary dyslexic, it lasts a lifetime.

After all these years my children are grown. They are all doing well—and I have lived to see my own hereditary dyslexia as an attribute. I look to our future with joy and anticipation. For me, man is a newcomer in the universe. Each human is unique. Yet all are so much alike that we can, to this day, readily understand and perhaps agree with a Chinese poet, writing in the seventh century.

Tell me now, what should a man want
But to sit alone, sipping his cup of wine?
I should like to have visitors come and discuss philosophy
And not have the tax-collector coming to collect taxes
My three sons married into good families
Then I could jog through a happy five-score years
And at the end, need no Paradise.

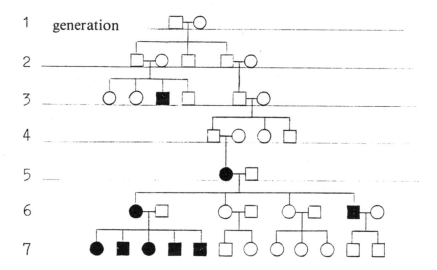

The inheritance of the hereditary dyslexic trait through seven
generations! The circles refer to females, the squares to males.
Two symbols joined directly by a horizontal line represent a
marriage, and the children are shown on the next line below,
with the birth order from left to right. Those individuals
showing the trait are indicated by a solid symbol.

# RESOURCES

1.  The Orton Dyslexia Society
    724 York Road
    Baltimore, Maryland 21204
    (301) 296-0232

2.  The Association for Children with Learning Disabilities
    4156 Library Road
    Pittsburgh, Pennsylvania 15234
    (412) 341-1515

3.  National Library Service for the Blind and Physically
    Handicapped
    Reference Section
    Library of Congress
    1291 Taylor Street, N.W.
    Washington, D.C. 20542
    (202) 287-5104

4.  The Frost School
    4915 Aspen Hill Road
    Rockville, Maryland 20853
    (301) 933-3451


The list which follows is taken from *Directory of Facilities and Services for the Learning Disabled, Tenth Edition*, published by Academic Therapy Publications, 20 Commercial Boulevard, Novato, California 94947. © 1983, Academic Therapy Publications, Inc. It is used with their permission.

Birmingham Educational Services
85 Bagby Drive
Birmingham, Alabama 35209
(205) 942-4008

Montgomery Dyslexia Foundation, Inc.
2229 Allendale Road
Montgomery, Alabama 36111
(205) 265-2840

Center for Neurodevelopmental Studies, Inc.
8621 N. Third Street
Phoenix, Arizona 85020
(602) 956-4214

New Way School
4140 N. Miller Road
Scottsdale, Arizona 85252
(602) 946-9112

A Learning Place
6472 Moraga Avenue
Oakland, California 94611
(415) 531-2500

Arena School
1123 Court Street
San Rafael, California 94901
(415) 453-3575

Center for Perceptual Development
2240 5th Avenue
San Diego, California 92101
(619) 233-6654

Dyslexia Counseling Center
1799 Old Bayshore Highway
Burlingame, California 94010
(415) 692-8990

Marianne Frostig Center of Educational Therapy
2495 E. Mountain Street
Pasadena, California 91104
(213) 791-1255

The Learning Center
Dominican College
San Rafael, California 94901
(415) 457-4440

Denver Academy
235 South Sherman
Denver, Colorado 80209
(303) 777-5870

Havern Center, Inc.
4000 South Wadsworth
Littleton, Colorado 80123
(303) 986-4587

Devereux in Connecticut
2 Sabbaday Lane
Washington, Connecticut 06793
(203) 868-7377

Villa Maria Education Center
159 Sky Meadow Drive
Stamford, Connecticut 06903
(203) 322-5886

Turning Point Children's Home, Inc.
698 Old Baltimore Pike
Newark, Delaware 19702
(302) 731-1137

George Washington University Reading Center
2201 G Street, N.W.
Washington, D.C. 20015
(202) 686-1774

Academic Achievement Center
7016 N. Donald Avenue
Tampa, Florida 33614
(813) 932-3731

Reading-Math Place
4301 32nd Street West
Bradenton, Florida 33507
(813) 756-3764

Woodland Hall Academy
Dyslexia Research Institute, Inc.
4745 Centerville Road
Tallahassee, Florida 32308
(904) 893-2216

Devereux in Georgia
1980 Stanley Road, N.W.
Kennesaw, Georgia 30144
(404) 427-0147

The Howard School, Inc.
436 Forrest Hill Road
Macon, Georgia 31210
(912) 477-8111

Assets School
Box 106
Pearl Harbor, Hawaii 96860
(808) 423-1720

Success Learning Programs
1061 Maunawili Road
Kailua, Hawaii 96734
(808) 261-0017

Brehm Preparatory School
1245 East Grand Avenue
Carbondale, Illinois 62901
(618) 457-0371

Chicago Clinic for Child Development
1525 East 53rd Street
Chicago, Illinois 60615
(312) 241-5771

Rosary College Educational Evaluation Center
7900 West Division Street
River Forest, Illinois 60305
(312) 366-2590

Strauss Learning Center
6214 Morenci Trail
Indianapolis, Indiana 46268
(317) 299-4331

Institute of Logopedics
2400 Jardine Drive
Wichita, Kansas 67219
(316) 262-8271

Midwest Reading & Dyslexia Clinic
8005 West 110th Street
Overland Park, Kansas 66210
(913) 341-3006

The de Paul School, Inc.
1925 Duker Avenue
Louisville, Kentucky 40205
(502) 459-6131

Ursuline-Pitt School
10715 Ward Avenue
Anchorage, Kentucky 40223

The Advancement School
206 Midway Drive
New Orleans, Louisiana 70123
(504) 737-5090

St. Bernard Developmental Center
3114 Paris Road
Chalmette, Louisiana 70043
(504) 279-5427

Center for Unique Learners
401 East Jefferson Street
Rockville, Maryland 20850
(301) 424-0250

Innovative Learning Center
1461 Old Annapolis Road
Arnold, Maryland 21012
(301) 974-1090

Devereux in Massachusetts
Two Miles Road
Rutland, Massachusetts 01543
(617) 886-4746

Linden Hill School
South Mountain Road
Northfield, Massachusetts 01360
(413) 498-2167

Riverview School
Route 6A
East Sandwich, Massachusetts 02537
(617) 888-0489

Camp Niobe
18443 Muirland
Detroit, Michigan 48221
(313) 796-2018

Neuro-Education Center
William Beaumont Hospital
3203 Coolidge Highway
Royal Oak, Michigan 48072
(313) 288-2332

West Side Family Mental Health Clinic
4025 West Main Street
Kalamazoo, Michigan 49007
(616) 381-2626

LDA Reading & Math Clinic
2344 Nicollet Avenue South
Minneapolis, Minnesota 55404
(612) 871-9011

The Groves Learning Center
3200 Highway 100
St. Louis Park, Minnesota 55416
(612) 920-6377

Merriam Park Vision Center
366 North Prior
St. Paul, Minnesota 55104
(612) 645-8124

The Churchill School
7501 Maryland Avenue
St. Louis, Missouri 63105
(314) 721-1224

Diagnosis & Intervention
4101 Oak
Kansas City, Missouri 64110
(816) 561-3285

Occupational Therapy Department
Research Medical Center
2316 East Meyer Boulevard
Kansas City, Missouri 64132
(816) 276-4147

Crotched Mountain Rehabilitation Center
Greenfield, New Hampshire 03047
(603) 547-3311

New England Trade & Technical Institute
750 Massabesic Street
Manchester, New Hampshire 03103
(603) 669-1231

Center School
46 Washington Valley Road
Warren, New Jersey 07060
(201) 356-5196

The Community School of Bergen County, Inc.
20 Booth Avenue
Englewood, New Jersey 07631
(201) 567-3630

de Paul Learning Center of Central Jersey
P. O. Box 1116
Edison, New Jersey 08817
(201) 985-0955

Devereux Deerhaven
Pottersville Road
Chester, New Jersey 07930
(201) 879-4500

The Wilson School
271 Boulevard
Mountain Lakes, New Jersey 07046
(201) 334-0181

Brush Ranch School
P. O. Box 2450
Santa Fe, New Mexico 87501
(505) 757-8772

Brooklyn Community Counseling Center
1592 Flatbush Avenue
Brooklyn, New York 11210
(212) 859-5522

Center for Reading and Learning Development
257 Lexington Avenue
New York, New York 10016
(212) 340-6284

Developmental Learning Program
Education Assistance Center
382 Main Street
Port Washington, New York 11050
(516) 883-3006

The Hallen School
1310 Harrison Avenue
Mamaroneck, New York 10543
(914) 381-2006

Program for Learning Disabled College Students
Adelphi University
Garden City, New York 11530
(516) 663-1006

The Winston Preparatory School
4 West 76th Street
New York, New York 10023
(212) 496-8400

Mary Dore School
108 Bradford Drive
Charlotte, North Carolina 28208
(704) 394-2341

Hill Learning Development Center
3130 Pickett Road
Durham, North Carolina 27705
(919) 489-7464

The Learning Center
16 First Avenue N.E.
Hickory, North Carolina 28601
(704) 328-5326

ACLD Learning Center
201 Wick Avenue
Youngstown, Ohio 44503
(216) 746-0604

The Educational Clinic, Inc.
867 South James Road
Columbus, Ohio 43227
(614) 236-1604

The Olympus Center
38 East Hollister Street
Cincinnati, Ohio 45219
(513) 621-4606

Townsend Learning Center
210 Bell Street
Chagrin Falls, Ohio 44022
(216) 247-8300

Jordan Diagnostic Center
5700 North Portland
Oklahoma City, Oklahoma 73112
(405) 946-3033

Timberridge Clinical School
6001 North Classen Boulevard
Oklahoma City, Oklahoma 73118
(405) 848-3518

The Children's Program
Good Samaritan Hospital & Medical Center
2215 N.W. Northrup
Portland, Oregon 97210
(503) 229-7220

Tree of Learning High School
9000 S.W. Beaverton Highway
Portland, Oregon 97225
(503) 297-2336

Allegheny Chapter—ACLD
5244 Clarwin Avenue
Pittsburgh, Pennsylvania 15229
(412) 931-7400

Devereux in Pennsylvania
19 South Waterloo
Devon, Pennsylvania 19333
(215) 964-3000

The Learning Center
444 East College Avenue
State College, Pennsylvania 16801
(814) 234-3450

Martha Lloyd School, Inc.
West Main Street
Troy, Pennsylvania 16947
(717) 297-2185
The Pathway School
Box 18
Audubon, Pennsylvania 19407
(215) 277-0660

Springdale School
50 Springdale Drive
Camden, South Carolina 29020
(803) 432-1791

Trident Academy, Inc.
P. O. Box 804
Mt. Pleasant, South Carolina 29464
(803) 884-7046

Bodine School
2432 Yester Oaks Drive
Germantown, Tennessee 38138
(901) 754-1800

Institute of Learning Research
3710 North Natchez
Nashville, Tennessee 37211
(615) 834-7832

Amarillo College Access Center
Box 447
Amarillo, Texas 79178
(806) 376-5111

The Briarwood School
12207 Whittington Drive
Houston, Texas 77077
(713) 493-1070

Crisman Preparatory School
2455 North Eastman Road
Longview, Texas 75601
(214) 758-9741

Devereux Center—Texas
P. O. Box 2666
Victoria, Texas 77902
(512) 575-8271

Preston Hollow Presbyterian School
9800 Preston Road
Dallas, Texas 75230
(214) 368-3886

Starpoint School
Texas Christian University
Fort Worth, Texas 76129
(817) 921-7141

Learning Problems Clinic
401 12th Avenue
Salt Lake City, Utah 84103
(801) 521-1693

Mountain West Clinic for Neuro-therapy
1544 South 325 West
Orem, Utah 84057
(801) 226-8111

Brattleboro Retreat
75 Linden Street
Brattleboro, Vermont 05301
(802) 257-7785

Winston L. Prouty Center
2 Oak Street
Brattleboro, Vermont 05301
(802) 257-7852

Vermont Achievement Center
88 Park Street
Rutland, Vermont 05701
(802) 775-2395

The Achievement Center
615 North Jefferson Street
Roanoke, Virginia 24016
(703) 982-0128

Charlottesville Center for Dyslexia
170 Rugby Road
Charlottesville, Virginia 22903
(804) 977-2010

Oakland School
Oakland Farm
Boyd Tavern, Virginia 22947
(804) 293-8965

Oakwood School
Children's Achievement Center
7210 Braddock Road
Annandale, Virginia 22003
(703) 941-5788

Eastside Educational Services, Inc.
10909 N.E. 4th
Bellevue, Washington 98004
(206) 455-2778

Sensory Integration Services
621 1/2 North Pine Street
Tacoma, Washington 98406
(206) 272-2870

Coleman Hatfield
315 White & Browning Building
Logan, West Virginia 25601
(304) 752-4694

Comprehensive Child Care Center
1836 South Avenue
La Crosse, Wisconsin 54601
(608) 782-7300

Eau Claire Academy
P. O. Box 1168
Eau Claire, Wisconsin 54702
(715) 834-6681

Foothills Academy
2312 18th Street, N.W.
Calgary, Alberta T2M 3T5
Canada
(403) 284-4617

MACLD Lions Learning Center
804 Preston Avenue
Winnipeg, Manitoba R3G 2O3
Canada
(204) 783-7049

Sunburst Educational Consulting Services
9 Negus Place
Yellowknife, Northwest Territory X1A 2P7
Canada
(403) 920-2546

Reinex Centre
143 Lakeshore Road East
Oakville, Ontario L6J 1H3
Canada
(416) 844-3240

Tomatis Centre
1121 Bellamy Road
Scarborough, Ontario M1H 3B9
Canada
(416) 431-5584

Tutorial & Educational Assistance
3118 Windwood Drive
Mississauga, Ontario L5N 2K5
Canada
(416) 826-2184

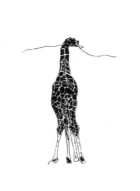

# BIBLIOGRAPHY

Allen, George. *The Human Spirit*. London: Ruskin House, 1960.

Bateson, Gregory. *Mind and Nature: A Necessary Unity*. New York: E. P. Dutton, 1979.

Bell, E. T. *Men of Mathematics: The Lives and Achievements of the Great Mathematicians from Zeno to Poincare*. New York: Simon & Schuster, 1937.

Berdyaev, Nikolai Aleksandrovich. *Slavery and Freedom*. New York: Charles Scribner's Sons, 1944.

——— *Truth and Revelation*. New York: Collier Books, 1962.

Bergson, Henri. *A Study in Metaphysics: The Creative Mind*. Totowa, NJ: Littlefield, Adams & Co., 1965.

Biermann, M. "Dyslexia Still Cannot Be Properly Defined." *German Tribune*, April 10, 1977.

Bronowski, J. *The Identity of Man*. New York: Natural History Press, 1966.

Buber, Martin. *Eclipse of God*. New York: Harper & Row, Publishers, Inc./Torchbooks, 1961.

——— *Good and Evil*. New York: Charles Scribner's Sons, 1952.

——— *I and Thou*, translated by R. G. Smith. New York: Charles Scribner's Sons, 1958.

——— *Two Types of Faith*. New York: Harper & Row, Publishers, Inc./Torchbooks, 1961.

Campbell, Joseph. *The Hero with a Thousand Faces*. Princeton, NJ: Princeton University Press, 1949.

Capra, Fritjof. *The Tao of Physics*. Boulder, CO: Shambhala Publications Inc., 1975.

Cirot, J. E. *A Dictionary of Symbols*, translated from the Spanish by J. Sage. New York: Philosophical Library, 1967.

Clark, Ronald W. *Einstein: The Life and Times.* New York: World Publishing Company, 1971.

Corballis, M. C., and I. L. Beale. "On Telling Left from Right." *Scientific American*, vol. 224, no. 3, p. 96. March, 1971.

Cousins, Norman. *Anatomy of an Illness.* New York: W. W. Norton & Co., 1979.

Critchley, MacDonald. *Dyslexia Defined: The Dyslexic Child.* Springfield, IL: Charles C. Thomas, Publishers, 1978.

Croce, Benedetto. *Aesthetic.* Darby, PA: Folcroft Library Editions, 1919.

Dantzig, Tobias. *Number: The Language of Science.* New York: Macmillan Publishing Company/The Free Press, 1967.

Dostoevski, Feodor M. *The Brothers Karamazov.* New York: The New American Library/Signet Books, 1958.

Durant, Will. *The Story of Philosophy.* New York: Simon & Schuster, 1926.

"Dyslexia: A Hemispheric Explanation." *Science News*, January 22, 1977.

Einstein, Albert. *Essays in Science.* New York: Philosophical Library, 1934.

——— *Ideas and Opinions, a Mathematician's Mind.* New York: Dell Publishing Company, 1976.

——— "Letter to Jacques Hadamard." *The Creative Process.* Berkeley, CA: University of California Press, 1952.

——— *Out of My Later Years.* New York: Philosophical Library, 1950.

——— *Relativity: The Special and General Theory.* New York: Crown Publishers Inc., 1971.

Ferguson, Marilyn. *The Brain Revolution.* New York: Taplinger Publishing Company, 1973.

Frankl, Viktor. *Man's Search for Meaning*. New York: Pocket Books, 1963.

Fromm, Erich. *The Art of Loving*. New York: Harper & Row, Publishers, Inc., 1956.

——— *You Shall Be as Gods*. New York: Holt, Rinehart & Winston, 1966.

Fuller, R. Buckminster. *I Seem to Be a Verb*. New York: Bantam Books, 1969.

Gazzaniga, M. S. "The Split Brain in Man." *Scientific American*, vol. 225, p. 24. August, 1967.

Geschwind, N. *Anatomical Evolution and the Human Brain*. Bulletin of the Orton Dyslexia Society, vol. XXII. Baltimore, MD, 1972.

——— *Asymmetries of the Brain: New Developments*. Bulletin of the Orton Dyslexia Society, vol. XXIX. Baltimore, MD, 1979.

——— and W. Levitsky. "The Human Brain: Left-Right Asymmetries in Temporal Speech Region." *Science*, vol. 161, pp. 186-187. 1968.

Ghiselin, Brewster. *The Creative Process*. Berkeley, CA: University of California Press, 1952.

Hall, Edward T. *Beyond Culture*. New York: Doubleday & Co., 1976.

——— *The Silent Language*. New York: Doubleday & Co., 1959.

Hallgren, Bertil. *Specific Dyslexia, "Congenital Word-Blindness": A Clinical and Genetic Study*. Stockholm, 1950.

Hammarskjold, Dag. *Markings*. New York: Alfred A. Knopf, 1965.

Heard, Gerald. *Pain, Sex, and Time*. London: Harper & Row, Publisher, Inc., 1939.

Hubben, William. *Four Prophets of Our Destiny: Dostoevsky, Kierkegaard, Nietzsche, and Kafka*. London: Collier-Macmillan, 1962.

Illich, Ivan. *Celebration of Awareness.* New York: Doubleday & Co., 1970.

James, William. *The Varieties of Religious Experience.* New York: Longmans, Green, 1902.

Jaynes, Julian. *The Origin of Consciousness in the Breakdown of the Bicameral Mind.* Boston: Houghton Mifflin Co., 1976.

Jung, Carl G. *Man and His Symbols.* New York: Doubleday & Co., 1964.

——— *Modern Man in Search of a Soul.* 1933.

——— *Psyche & Symbols.* New York: Doubleday & Co., 1958.

——— *Psychology and Religion: West and East.* Princeton, NJ: Princeton University Press, 1958.

——— *The Undiscovered Self.* New York: The New American Library, 1957.

Kazantzakis, Nikos. *The Last Temptation of Christ.* New York: Simon & Schuster, 1960.

Kierkegaard, Soren. *Fear and Trembling* and *The Sickness Unto Death.* Princeton, NJ: Princeton University Press, 1941.

——— *Purity of Heart.* New York: Harper & Row, Publishers, Inc./Torchbooks, 1938.

Knud, Hermann. *Reading Disability: A Medical Study of Word-Blindness and Related Handicaps.* Springfield, IL: Charles C. Thomas, Publisher, 1959.

Lamb, H. *Genghis Khan: Emperor of All Men.* New York: Bantam Books, 1953.

Landis, Paul., editor. *Four Famous Greek Plays.* New York: Random House/Modern Library, 1929.

Lecomte du Nouy. *Human Destiny.* New York: Longmans, Green, 1947.

Lee, J. R. "The Triune Brain." *Somatics*, vol. II, p. 17. Novato, CA, 1980.

Lynch, William F. *The Images of Hope: Imagination as Healer of the Hopeless*. Notre Dame, IN: University of Notre Dame Press, 1974.

McLuhan, Marshall. *The Gutenberg Galaxy*. Toronto: University of Toronto Press, 1962.

――― *The Medium Is the Message*. New York: Bantam Books, 1967.

――― *Understanding Media: The Extensions of Man*. New York: The New American Library, 1964.

――― "What Television Is Doing to Us and Why." *The Washington Post*, May 15, 1971.

Masland, Richard L. *The Advantages of Being Dyslexic*. Bulletin of the Orton Dyslexia Society, vol. XXVI, p. 10. Baltimore, MD, 1976.

Maslow, Abraham. *Religions, Values, and Peak Experiences*. New York: The Viking Press, 1970.

――― *Toward a Psychology of Being*. New York: D. Van Nostrand Co., 1968.

Menninger, Karl. *The Human Mind*. New York: The Literary Guild, 1930.

Ornstein, Robert. *The Psychology of Consciousness*. New York: Penguin Books, 1972.

Otto, Rudolf. *The Idea of the Holy*. New York: Oxford University Press, 1958.

Overstreet, Harry. *The Mature Mind*. New York: W. W. Norton & Co., 1949.

――― *The Mind Alive*. New York: W. W. Norton & Co., 1954.

Pollack, Cecelia. *Neuropsychological Aspects of Reading and Writing*. Bulletin of the Orton Dyslexia Society, vol. XXVI, p. 19. Baltimore, MD, 1976.

Rawson, Margaret B. *Developmental Language Disability*. Baltimore, MD: The Johns Hopkins University Press, 1968.

――― *The Self Concept and the Cycle of Growth*. Bulletin of the Orton Dyslexia Society, vol. XXIV. Baltimore, MD, 1974.

Riesman, David. *The Lonely Crowd*. New Haven, CT: Yale University Press, 1950.

Rockefeller, Nelson A. *TV Guide*, 1976.

Rome, H. D. *The Psychiatric Aspects of Dyslexia*. Bulletin of the Orton Dyslexia Society, vol. XXI. Baltimore, MD, 1971.

Rozin, P., Poritsky, S., and R. Sotsky. "American Children with Reading Problems Can Easily Learn to Read English Represented by Chinese Characters." *Science*, vol. 171. March, 1971.

Russell, Bertrand. *The ABC of Relativity*. New York: The New American Library, 1958.

Sartre, Jean-Paul. *Of Human Freedom*. New York: Philosophical Library, 1966.

——— *The Words*. New York: George Braziller Inc., 1964.

Schrodinger, Erwin. *What Is Life? and Other Scientific Essays*. New York: Doubleday & Co., 1956.

Schweitzer, Albert. *The Quest of the Historical Jesus*. New York: Macmillan Publishing Co., 1968.

Simpson, Eileen. *Reversals: A Personal Account of Victory over Dyslexia*. New York: Washington Square Press/Pocket Books, 1981.

Sladen, Brenda. *Some Genetic Aspects of Dyslexia*. Bulletin of the Orton Dyslexia Society, vol. XXII. Baltimore, MD, 1972.

Sperry, R. W. "Cerebral Organization and Behavior." *Science*, vol. 133, p. 1749. June 2, 1961.

——— "Great Cerebral Commissure." *Scientific American*, vol. 210, p. 42. January, 1964.

——— "Left-Brain, Right-Brain." *Saturday Review*, vol. II, p. 50. August 9, 1975.

Strong, L. *Language Disability in the Hispano-American Child*. Bulletin of the Orton Dyslexia Society, vol. XXIII. Baltimore, MD, 1973.

Teilhard de Chardin, Pierre. *The Divine Milieu*. New York: Harper & Row, Publishers, Inc., 1960.

——— *Human Energy*. New York: Harcourt Brace Jovanovich, 1969.

——— *The Phenomenon of Man*. New York: Harper & Row, Publishers, Inc., 1961.

Thompson, Lloyd. *The International Scene*. Bulletin of the Orton Dyslexia Society, vol. XXIII, p. 28. Baltimore, MD, 1973.

——— *Language Disabilities in Men of Eminence*. Bulletin of the Orton Dyslexia Society, vol. XIX. Baltimore, MD, 1969.

Tillich, Paul. *The Courage to Be*. New Haven, CT: Yale University Press, 1952.

——— "The Meaning of Joy." In the anthology *The Human Spirit*, edited by Whit Burnett. London: Allen & Unwin, 1960.

——— *The New Being*. New York: Charles Scribner's Sons, 1955.

Unamuno y Jugo, Miguel de. *The Agony of Christianity*. New York: Frederick Ungar Publishing Co., 1960.

——— *Tragic Sense of Life*. New York: Dover Publications Inc., 1941.

Waley, Arthur. *Translations from the Chinese*. New York: Alfred A. Knopf, 1941.

West, C. *Communism and the Theologians*. Philadelphia: The Westminster Press, 1958.

Wiener, Norbert. *Cybernetics*. Cambridge, MA: The MIT Press, 1961.

Witelson, Sandra. "Developmental Dyslexia: Two Right Hemispheres and None Left." *Science*, vol. 195, pp. 309-311. January, 1977.